Table of Contents

Introduction
Chapter 1: Understanding Veganism
Chapter 2: Health Benefits
Chapter 3: Making the Transition
Chapter 4: Long Term Nutritional Considerations
Chapter 5: Beyond the Vegan Diet
Chapter 6: Resources
Chapter 7: Sample Vegan Meal Plans
Chapter 8: Continuing Your Vegan Journey
Appendix

Disclaimer

Nothing in this guide or included as part of this information, should be construed as an attempt to offer, or render a medical opinion or otherwise engage in the practice of medicine.

This guide is not intended to diagnose, treat, or cure any illness. Please contact a medical professional for advice.

All content is subject to copyright and may not be reproduced in any form without express written consent from the author.

Introduction

Hi, I'm Kristina, and thanks for purchasing my eBook. Over the past ten years, I made several major lifestyle changes that made a significant impact on my body, skin, and overall health. There has been a remarkable change within me, and it has radiated out so much that my friends and family have taken notice. People who have known me throughout this change have commented that I look great, and have been asking me what I did, what my secret is. The answer is complex, so I decided to put it into a book and share it with the rest of the world.

First, I would like to make a disclaimer that I am not a doctor, and I do not play one on the internet. The information in this eBook are my own thoughts and opinions based on my real-life experience. Please consult with your doctor before making any changes to your current diet and exercise program.

Second, I want to iterate that my goal is not to be skinny or lose weight. My goal is to make good choices daily, to have optimal health, and feel good about myself knowing that I am giving it my best effort. This is not a quick fix, but a lifestyle change that I practice every day. Some weeks are great, and I feel awesome, but some weeks are not so great, and I must reassess what my goals are and why something is not working. It could take weeks, months, even years for these habits to transform your life. There is a lot of self-love and self-acceptance involved in this practice as well. After all these years of healthy eating, I still have stretch marks from having kids that used to embarrass me. Now I am proud of what my body has gone through, and its strength and capability to bring four healthy children into this amazing world. You too can have that pride in your body, without fitting into whatever the rest of the world declares to be "perfect." Loving yourself and taking care of your body are the first steps in changing your life and living to your full potential.

Keep an open mind, and do not worry if you fall off track. It can be frustrating. but do not beat yourself up over it, learn from how you fell off, put processes in place so it does not happen again, and keep trying!

Peace and Love.

Kristina Reslin

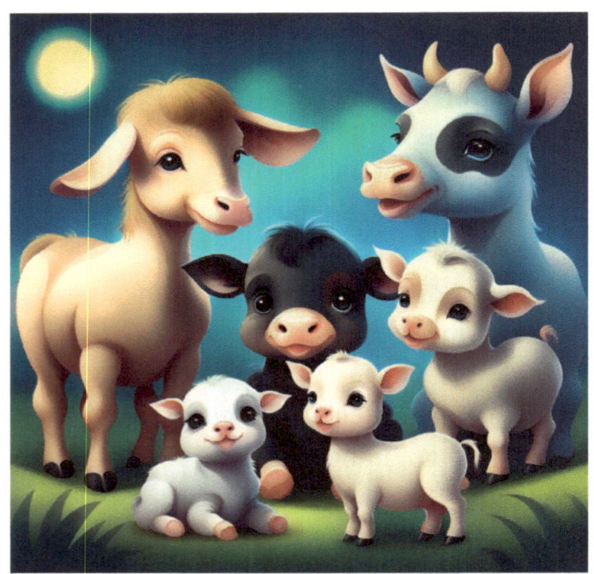

In a world where dietary choices can have profound implications for our health, the environment, and the welfare of animals, the concept of veganism stands as a testament to the power of individual choices to effect positive change. Veganism, a lifestyle that abstains from all forms of animal exploitation, has emerged as a compelling response to the ethical, environmental, and health concerns that have become increasingly prominent in our global consciousness.

At the heart of veganism lies a profound ethical commitment – a recognition of the moral duty to protect the rights and well-being of animals. Veganism asserts that sentient beings, regardless of their species, deserve to live free from suffering and exploitation. Ethical vegans choose to boycott industries that profit from animal suffering, such as factory farming, fur production, and animal testing. Their actions reflect a belief in the intrinsic value of all life and a dedication to fostering a more compassionate world. The environmental consequences of our dietary choices have never been more apparent. Animal agriculture, a major driver of deforestation, habitat loss, and greenhouse gas emissions, poses a significant threat to our planet's ecological balance. Choosing veganism is a powerful statement of environmental stewardship. It acknowledges the need to reduce our ecological footprint, conserve biodiversity, and mitigate climate change by opting for plant-based foods, which require fewer resources and produce fewer emissions.

Beyond its ethical and environmental merits, veganism offers substantial health benefits. Scientific research has shown that a well-balanced vegan diet can lower the risk of chronic diseases, such as heart disease, diabetes, and certain types of cancer. By prioritizing fruits, vegetables, whole grains, nuts, and legumes, vegans often enjoy improved cardiovascular health, lower cholesterol levels, and healthier body weights. The decision to go vegan, therefore, can be a transformative journey toward personal well-being and vitality.

As we embark on this exploration of veganism, we will delve deeper into these facets, unraveling the ethical, environmental, and health dimensions of this profound lifestyle choice. By the end of this journey, you will have a comprehensive understanding of not only why people choose veganism but also how you can make informed and empowered choices that align with your values and aspirations for a brighter, more compassionate, and sustainable future.

This book is for anyone considering a vegan lifestyle, Vegetarians looking to transition into veganism, or anyone just curious about plant-based diets. In this book we will cover what Veganism entails, the health benefits, making the transition, How to Build your Vegan Pantry, Eating out and Traveling, Maintaining a Balanced Diet, and of course, Resources and Recipes.

Chapter 1: Understanding Veganism

Being vegan is a lifestyle and dietary choice that involves abstaining from the use of all animal products, both in one's diet and in other aspects of life. Here's a comprehensive explanation of what it means to be vegan.

At its core, veganism pertains to food choices. A vegan diet excludes all animal-derived ingredients, which means not consuming:

Meat: This includes beef, pork, poultry, lamb, and any other animal flesh.
Dairy Products: Such as milk, cheese, butter, and yogurt, which are produced from the milk of cows, goats, or other mammals.
Eggs: Vegans do not eat eggs or foods containing eggs.
Fish and Seafood: All types of fish and seafood are off-limits to vegans.
Honey: Some vegans choose to avoid honey because it is produced by bees.
Gelatin: Derived from animal collagen, gelatin is found in many food products and is avoided by vegans.

Veganism is driven by ethical considerations. Vegans believe in the inherent value and rights of all sentient beings, regardless of species. They are against the exploitation, suffering, and killing of animals for human purposes, including food, clothing, entertainment, and scientific experimentation.

Many vegans also adopt this lifestyle due to environmental reasons. They recognize that the animal agriculture industry is a major contributor to deforestation, habitat destruction, water pollution, and greenhouse gas emissions. By choosing plant-based foods, vegans aim to reduce their ecological footprint and promote a more sustainable planet.

While not all vegans choose this lifestyle for health reasons, many enjoy its health benefits. A well-balanced vegan diet can be rich in fruits, vegetables, whole grains, nuts, and legumes, which are generally associated with lower risks of chronic diseases like heart disease, diabetes, and certain types of cancer. Vegans often have lower cholesterol levels and healthier body weights compared to omnivores.

Veganism extends beyond dietary choices. Many vegans also make conscious decisions in other areas of life, such as clothing and personal care products. They avoid clothing made from animal materials like fur, leather, and wool, and they choose cruelty-free, vegan-friendly cosmetics and toiletries. Some vegans also refuse to support industries that use animals for entertainment, like circuses and marine parks.

Veganism often involves advocacy and activism to promote animal welfare, environmental conservation, and healthier eating habits. Vegans may engage in activities such as sharing information, participating in protests, and supporting organizations that align with their values.

In essence, being vegan means aligning one's lifestyle and choices with a set of values that prioritize compassion for animals, sustainability, and personal health. It involves making conscious decisions to avoid the use of animal products and to promote a more ethical, eco-friendly, and humane way of living.

But What is the Difference Between Veganism and Simply Being Vegetarian?

Veganism and vegetarianism are both dietary choices that involve abstaining from consuming certain animal products, but they differ in the extent to which they exclude these products:

Vegans do not consume any animal products whatsoever, both in their diet and in other aspects of life. This includes not only meat but also all animal-derived foods like dairy, eggs, and honey. Vegans avoid all animal meats (beef, pork, poultry, etc.), seafood, dairy products (milk, cheese, butter, yogurt), eggs, honey, and any other foods containing these ingredients. While health considerations may also play a role, many vegans choose this lifestyle primarily for ethical and environmental reasons. They believe in the inherent value of all sentient beings and seek to minimize harm to animals and the planet. Beyond diet, vegans often extend their ethical choices to other areas of life. They may avoid wearing clothing made from animal materials (leather, fur, wool) and using products tested on animals. They also reject forms of entertainment that exploit animals.

Vegetarians do not consume the flesh of animals but may include some animal-derived products in their diet, such as dairy and eggs. The extent of these inclusions can vary among different types of vegetarians.

Lacto-Ovo Vegetarian: Excludes meat and seafood but includes dairy products (lacto) and eggs (ovo).
Lacto-Vegetarian: Excludes meat, seafood, and eggs but includes dairy products.
Ovo-Vegetarian: Excludes meat, seafood, and dairy products but includes eggs.
Pescatarian: Excludes meat and poultry but includes seafood.
Vegetarians may have various reasons for their dietary choices, including ethical concerns about animal slaughter (especially in the case of lacto-vegetarians and ovo-vegetarians), environmental considerations, and health motivations.

While vegetarianism primarily deals with diet, some vegetarians may also extend their ethical choices to other aspects of life, similar to vegans. However, this is less common among vegetarians compared to vegans.

In summary, the key difference between veganism and vegetarianism lies in the exclusion of animal products from the diet. Vegans exclude all animal products, including dairy, eggs, and honey, while vegetarians may include some of these products based on their specific type of vegetarianism. Ethical and environmental concerns are often stronger motivators for vegans, whereas various factors, including ethics, health, and environmental considerations, influence different types of vegetarians.

History of Veganism

The development of veganism as a lifestyle has been marked by significant milestones over the years. In 1944, Donald Watson and Elsie Shrigley, two members of the Leicester Vegetarian Society in England, formed The Vegan Society. They coined the term "vegan" by taking the first three and last two letters of "vegetarian" to represent a lifestyle that abstains from all animal products. This marked the formal beginning of the vegan movement. The Vegan Society published the first issue of "The Vegan News," in 1944 which was the world's first vegan magazine. It provided a platform for sharing information, recipes, and resources related to veganism. Inspired by The Vegan Society in the UK, vegan societies were founded in various countries, including the United States and Australia, during the 1940s and 1950s. These organizations played a crucial role in spreading the principles of veganism globally.

Philosopher Peter Singer's book "Animal Liberation" in 1975 contributed significantly to the modern animal rights movement. It raised awareness about the ethical treatment of animals and influenced many individuals to consider veganism as a response to animal suffering. During the 1980s and 1990s, vegan activism gained momentum with the formation of organizations like People for the Ethical Treatment of Animals (PETA). These groups conducted high-profile campaigns, protests, and educational initiatives to promote veganism and animal rights.

Scientific research on plant-based nutrition and its health benefits became more prominent in the late 20th century. Studies highlighting the advantages of a vegan diet for reducing the risk of chronic diseases, such as heart disease and certain cancers, contributed to the growth of veganism. The 21st century saw an increase in vegan celebrities and influencers using their platforms to promote veganism. High-profile figures like musicians, actors, athletes, and chefs have helped popularize the lifestyle and its benefits. The availability of vegan products, including plant-based meat substitutes, dairy alternatives, and vegan-friendly packaged foods, has grown exponentially in the 21st century. This accessibility has made it easier for people to transition to a vegan diet.

Documentaries such as "Forks Over Knives," "Cowspiracy," and "What the Health" have raised awareness about the health and environmental aspects of veganism. Media coverage of vegan-related topics has also played a role in spreading information about the lifestyle. Events like World Vegan Day (November 1st) and Veganuary (a campaign encouraging people to try veganism in January) have gained popularity worldwide. These initiatives help introduce people to veganism and provide resources and support.

These milestones, among others, have contributed to the growth and recognition of veganism as a lifestyle that encompasses ethical, environmental, and health considerations. Veganism has evolved from a relatively obscure movement to a global phenomenon with millions of adherents advocating for a more compassionate and sustainable world.

The Moral Arguments for Veganism

The food industry, sadly, is a business and their animals are a commodity. Pigs and hens are packed like sardines in cages, unable to move for the duration of their life, living in disease and fear. Laws have been put in place to protect these factory farms from whistle-blowers, and the brave people who document these atrocities live in fear of being prosecuted and jailed for informing the public about where their food comes from.

Working in the auto industry for most of my career, I noticed some huge ethical differences between the auto and food industry in the United States regarding transparency, consumer rights, and protecting the environment. In the auto industry, safety is the number one priority before profits. Several automotive assembly plants provide tours to the public and encourage their employees to speak up if there is a safety issue. Factory farms have never been open to the public, and it is illegal to film without the consent of the owner. One would think that an industry that makes a product that is vital to life- food- that absolute transparency would be mandated. However, it is the absolute opposite. People are being punished for speaking out and exposing factory farms, it has literally turned into the foxes protecting the henhouse.

In the United States, auto manufacturers have Corporate Average Fuel Economy (CAFÉ) regulations on cars and light trucks, to improve average fuel economy standards, and reduce energy consumption. Factory farms have no such regulations on energy consumption, or even regulations on the water that they pollute when disposing of animal waste. The EPA estimates that 11% of greenhouse gas emissions in the United States come from Agriculture, and the animal manure that is stored in lagoons releases methane and nitrous oxide, which is a more powerful greenhouse gas than carbon dioxide. It has been researched by author Denis Hayes, that "the amount of carbon dioxide that is given off per pound of beef, is in fact, greater, than burning a gallon of gasoline." This calculation considers the energy required to fertilize the fields, harvest the animal feed, and transportation just to feed the cow that ends up being slaughtered for beef.

If you are now wondering why the Farming industry has so much power to avoid regulations and silence protesters, let's follow the money. According to the Senate Office of Public Records, over $66 million dollars has been spent for 2017, as of the end of August, on Lobbying, and for this same time period, the automotive industry has spent a little over $26 million dollars on lobbying. During this research, I also found it interesting that the pharmaceutical industry had by far the highest dollar amount spent on lobbying, at $145 million dollars for the same time period. Could it be a racket in which the food industry creates our diseases, and the pharmaceutical industry develops the cures? This is my conspiracy theory, but it does make sense. Why would the food industry spend so much money to ensure privacy from the public. Doesn't the public have a right to know what they are feeding themselves and their children? And why can't the public be aware of what practices are being used in the journey from the factory to your plate?

I could write another book on the evils of factory farming, but I will leave you with this: Do you want to continue to support an industry that will turn around and sell you products from infected and diseased animals, pollute the air and water, and then prosecute anyone that stands up to them? I say, don't give them a cent, and eventually the Meat and Dairy industry will topple because of their bad karma.

Speaking of karma, my personal reason for not consuming dairy or cow's milk is as follows. Imagine you have just given birth to a child, and seconds later your child is being drug away from you, put in a box to be slaughtered. A machine is hooked up to your nipples and your milk is being stolen from you as you cry for your baby. All that negative energy from the cow's milk enters your body when you eat a piece of cheese pizza, or have a glass of milk, and the cycle of karma continues. By making ethical choices with the food you consume, you can stop the flow of negative energy into your life. This may sound like some hippy-dippy crap to you, but I can speak from experience that it has been true for me. After cutting cheese, eggs, and milk out of my diet, I have noticed that I no longer get sinus infections or tension headaches, and my body has never felt better. I have abundant amounts of positive energy, so much so, that I find myself writing an eBook to inform others of this wonderful process, while being a mother of four children and working full time. Miracles can and will start happening in your life as well.

Moral arguments for veganism are rooted in the belief that animals have inherent value and rights, and that it is morally wrong to exploit or harm them unnecessarily. Central to the moral argument for veganism is the concept of animal rights. Advocates argue that animals, like humans, have the right to live free from unnecessary suffering and exploitation. They assert that using animals for food, clothing, entertainment, or experimentation often involves cruel practices that violate these rights. Veganism is seen as a way to minimize harm and suffering inflicted on animals. Factory farming practices, in particular, are often criticized for confining animals in overcrowded, unsanitary conditions, subjecting them to stress, disease, and painful procedures like debeaking or tail docking.

Advocates argue that discrimination based on species, known as speciesism, is morally unjust. Just as it is wrong to discriminate against individuals based on their race, gender, or other characteristics, it is also wrong to discriminate against animals simply because they belong to a different species. Many moral arguments for veganism emphasize the importance of aligning one's moral values with one's actions. If one believes that causing unnecessary harm to animals is wrong, then adopting a vegan lifestyle is seen as a consistent way to live in accordance with those values.

Vegans argue that by choosing not to support industries that exploit animals, they reduce the economic demand for products derived from animals. This, in turn, can lead to a reduction in the production and suffering of animals in these industries. Some moral arguments for veganism also touch on environmental ethics. The livestock industry is a major contributor to environmental problems like deforestation, habitat destruction, and climate change. Advocates argue that by reducing or eliminating animal agriculture, one can contribute to a more sustainable and ethical use of resources. Veganism is often viewed as a form of ethical consumerism, where individuals make choices that align with their moral values. This includes supporting businesses and products that adhere to cruelty-free and sustainable practices.

Some advocates point out the moral implications of the global food system, where grains and resources that could feed humans are diverted to feed animals in factory farms. They argue that veganism can help address food inequity by using resources more efficiently. Veganism respects cultural diversity and individual choice while encouraging critical reflection on cultural practices that involve animal exploitation. It promotes a more inclusive and compassionate approach to food and lifestyle choices.

Moral arguments for veganism vary in their philosophical underpinnings, but they all share a fundamental concern for the well-being and ethical treatment of animals. Supporters of veganism believe that adopting a plant-based diet and lifestyle is a meaningful way to reduce harm to animals and promote a more compassionate and just world.

The role of animal agriculture in climate change is significant, as it contributes to several aspects of the climate crisis, including greenhouse gas emissions, deforestation, and habitat destruction. Here's a breakdown of how animal agriculture impacts climate change:

Greenhouse Gas Emissions:

Carbon Dioxide (CO2): Animal agriculture contributes to CO2 emissions through deforestation, as forests are often cleared to make way for livestock grazing and feed crop production. This results in the release of stored carbon from trees and soil.

Methane (CH4): Livestock, particularly cattle, produce methane during digestion through a process called enteric fermentation. Methane is a potent greenhouse gas, with a much higher heat-trapping potential than CO2 over the short term.

Nitrous Oxide (N2O): Animal waste and the application of synthetic fertilizers to grow animal feed crops release nitrous oxide, another potent greenhouse gas.

Large swaths of forests are cleared to create space for livestock grazing and to grow crops, such as soy and corn, used as animal feed. This deforestation not only releases stored carbon into the atmosphere but also reduces the Earth's capacity to absorb CO2, exacerbating climate change. The expansion of animal agriculture often leads to the conversion of diverse ecosystems into monoculture farms, which reduces biodiversity and further contributes to ecological imbalances. Animal agriculture consumes substantial amounts of water, from providing drinking water for livestock to irrigating feed crops. The water-intensive nature of this industry places stress on freshwater resources, which are essential for sustaining ecosystems and human populations. Overgrazing by livestock can lead to soil erosion and land degradation, reducing the land's ability to sequester carbon and support vegetation that helps mitigate climate change.

The disposal of animal waste in concentrated animal feeding operations (CAFOs) can lead to water pollution, as excess nutrients and pathogens can enter waterways, further contributing to environmental problems and negatively impacting aquatic ecosystems.

Animal agriculture is energy-intensive, involving the production of feed, transportation of animals, and processing of meat products. The associated fossil fuel use contributes to CO2 emissions and exacerbates the climate crisis. Climate change itself, driven in part by animal agriculture, can result in extreme weather events, shifts in precipitation patterns, and temperature increases that threaten food security. This can disproportionately affect vulnerable communities and regions dependent on agriculture.

Climate change can create feedback loops that further exacerbate environmental degradation. For example, as temperatures rise due to climate change, it can lead to more frequent and severe heat waves, which stress livestock and reduce their productivity, increasing the pressure on the industry to expand and intensify operations.

It's important to note that the impact of animal agriculture on climate change varies depending on factors such as production methods, livestock types, and land management practices. Sustainable and regenerative agricultural practices, as well as reducing meat consumption and shifting to plant-based diets, are considered key strategies to mitigate the climate impact of animal agriculture and address the broader climate crisis.

Chapter 2: Health Benefits

Overview of Essential Nutrients and Their Vegan Sources
A well-balanced vegan diet can provide all the essential nutrients your body needs for optimal health. Here is an overview of these nutrients and their vegan sources:

Protein:
Sources: Legumes (beans, lentils, chickpeas), tofu, tempeh, seitan, edamame, quinoa, nuts, seeds, and whole grains like brown rice and oats.

Calcium:
Sources: Fortified plant-based milk (soy, almond, rice, oat, etc.), fortified orange juice, tofu (if calcium-set), leafy greens (kale, collard greens, bok choy), and almonds.

Iron:
Sources: Legumes, tofu, quinoa, fortified cereals, pumpkin seeds, spinach, lentils, dried apricots, and cashews. Consuming iron-rich foods with vitamin C-rich foods enhances absorption.

Vitamin B12:
Sources: Fortified foods (plant-based milk, breakfast cereals, nutritional yeast), B12 supplements, or B12-fortified meat substitutes. Vitamin B12 is not naturally present in plant-based foods.

Omega-3 Fatty Acids:
Sources: Chia seeds, flaxseeds, hemp seeds, walnuts, and algae-based supplements (providing EPA and DHA, essential omega-3s).

Vitamin D:
Sources: Sunlight exposure triggers vitamin D synthesis in the skin. Vegans may consider vitamin D supplements, particularly in regions with limited sunlight.

Folate (Vitamin B9):
Sources: Dark leafy greens, lentils, chickpeas, asparagus, broccoli, and fortified cereals.

Zinc:
Sources: Legumes, whole grains, nuts (especially cashews and almonds), tofu, and seeds (pumpkin seeds).

Iodine:

Sources: Iodized salt, seaweed (but iodine content can vary, and excessive consumption is not recommended), and iodine-fortified foods.

Magnesium:
Sources: Nuts (almonds, cashews), seeds (pumpkin, sunflower), legumes, whole grains (oats, brown rice), leafy greens, and tofu.

Vitamin A (Beta-Carotene):
Sources: Orange and yellow fruits and vegetables (carrots, sweet potatoes, butternut squash), dark leafy greens (spinach, kale), and mangoes.

Vitamin E:
Sources: Nuts (almonds, hazelnuts), seeds (sunflower seeds, almonds), spinach, and broccoli.

Vitamin K:
Sources: Dark leafy greens (kale, collard greens, spinach), broccoli, Brussels sprouts, and green herbs like basil and parsley.

Phosphorus:
Sources: Legumes, nuts, seeds, whole grains, tofu, and tempeh.

Potassium:
Sources: Bananas, potatoes, sweet potatoes, oranges, spinach, and beans.

Selenium:
Sources: Brazil nuts (particularly high), whole grains, legumes, and tofu.

It's important for vegans to eat a variety of foods to ensure they get a wide range of nutrients. Planning balanced meals and, if necessary, considering fortified foods or supplements can help vegans meet their nutritional needs. Consulting a healthcare professional or registered dietitian can provide personalized guidance on achieving optimal nutrition on a vegan diet.

Common misconceptions about vegan nutrition can lead to concerns about inadequate nutrient intake. It's essential to address these misconceptions with accurate information:

Lack of Protein:
Misconception: People often assume that vegans cannot get enough protein because they don't consume animal products.
Reality: Plant-based sources like beans, lentils, tofu, tempeh, seitan, and quinoa provide ample protein. Most vegans can meet or exceed their protein needs with a well-balanced diet.

Calcium Deficiency:

Misconception: Vegans are at risk of calcium deficiency since they don't consume dairy products.

Reality: Plant-based sources like fortified plant milk, tofu, dark leafy greens, almonds, and calcium-set tofu can provide sufficient calcium. Additionally, some studies suggest that a lower intake of animal protein may lead to better calcium retention.

Vitamin B12:

Misconception: A vegan diet can naturally provide vitamin B12.

Reality: Vitamin B12 is not naturally present in plant-based foods. Vegans should rely on fortified foods or supplements to meet their B12 needs, as deficiency can have severe health consequences.

Iron Deficiency:

Misconception: Plant-based iron (non-heme iron) is not as absorbable as heme iron from animal products, leading to iron deficiency.

Reality: While non-heme iron is less readily absorbed, consuming vitamin C-rich foods alongside iron-rich foods can enhance absorption. Many vegans meet their iron needs by eating a varied diet, including lentils, beans, and leafy greens.

Omega-3 Fatty Acids:

Misconception: Vegans cannot get enough omega-3 fatty acids since they don't consume fish.

Reality: Plant-based sources like flaxseeds, chia seeds, hemp seeds, and walnuts provide alpha-linolenic acid (ALA), a type of omega-3 fatty acid. Vegans can also consider algae-based supplements for EPA and DHA, two other essential omega-3s.

Complete Proteins:

Misconception: Plant foods lack complete proteins, meaning they do not contain all essential amino acids.

Reality: While individual plant foods may not be complete proteins, eating a variety of plant-based foods throughout the day provides all essential amino acids. Combining foods like rice and beans or hummus and whole-grain pita can ensure protein completeness.

Inadequate Calories:

Misconception: A vegan diet lacks sufficient calories, leading to energy deficits.

Reality: With proper meal planning, vegans can meet their calorie needs. Whole grains, legumes, nuts, seeds, and healthy fats like avocados can provide ample calories.

Vegan Children's Nutrition:

Misconception: Vegan diets are unsuitable for children and can lead to growth and development issues.

Reality: Well-planned vegan diets can meet the nutritional needs of children. Paying attention to key nutrients like calcium, iron, vitamin B12, and vitamin D is crucial.

Low Nutrient Absorption:

Misconception: Plant-based diets are less nutrient-dense because they contain antinutrients that hinder nutrient absorption.

Reality: While some plant compounds may inhibit nutrient absorption, the overall nutrient density of a well-balanced vegan diet can be high. Cooking and food preparation methods can also help reduce antinutrient content.

Addressing these misconceptions and ensuring a varied, balanced vegan diet can help individuals meet their nutritional needs while enjoying the benefits of a plant-based lifestyle. Consulting a registered dietitian or healthcare professional can provide personalized guidance on vegan nutrition.

A vegan diet can reduce the risk of chronic diseases through various mechanisms related to its emphasis on plant-based foods and the avoidance of animal products. Here's how a vegan diet can contribute to a lower risk of chronic illnesses:

Reduced Saturated Fat and Cholesterol Intake:

A vegan diet eliminates or significantly reduces the intake of saturated fats and dietary cholesterol, which are primarily found in animal products. High consumption of these components is linked to heart disease.

Lower Blood Pressure:

Vegan diets tend to be high in potassium-rich foods like fruits and vegetables and low in sodium, which can help lower blood pressure. High blood pressure is a risk factor for heart disease and stroke.

Improved Blood Lipid Profile:

Vegan diets are associated with lower levels of total cholesterol, LDL cholesterol (the "bad" cholesterol), and triglycerides. These improvements in lipid profiles are protective against atherosclerosis and heart disease.

Weight Management:

Vegans often have a lower body mass index (BMI) compared to omnivores and vegetarians. Maintaining a healthy weight reduces the risk of obesity-related conditions such as type 2 diabetes, heart disease, and certain cancers.

Reduced Risk of Type 2 Diabetes:
Vegan diets are linked to a decreased risk of type 2 diabetes. High-fiber, low-fat plant foods can help regulate blood sugar levels and improve insulin sensitivity.

Improved Gut Health:
Vegan diets tend to be rich in dietary fiber from fruits, vegetables, whole grains, legumes, and nuts. This high fiber intake promotes a healthy gut microbiome, which has been associated with a reduced risk of various chronic diseases.

Antioxidant-Rich Foods:
A vegan diet includes a wide variety of antioxidant-rich foods such as fruits, vegetables, berries, nuts, and seeds. Antioxidants help combat oxidative stress and inflammation, which are underlying factors in chronic diseases.

Cancer Prevention:
Plant-based diets are associated with a lower risk of certain cancers, particularly colorectal, breast, and prostate cancers. The phytochemicals and fiber in plant foods play protective roles in reducing cancer risk.

Heart-Healthy Fats:
Vegans often consume heart-healthy fats, such as monounsaturated and polyunsaturated fats found in avocados, nuts, seeds, and olive oil. These fats can have a positive impact on heart health.

Lower Risk of Kidney Disease:
Plant-based diets may reduce the risk of kidney disease and slow its progression in individuals with pre-existing kidney conditions, in part due to reduced protein intake and improved blood pressure control.

Reduced Inflammation:
Plant-based diets are associated with lower levels of systemic inflammation, which is a contributing factor to many chronic diseases, including heart disease, diabetes, and certain autoimmune conditions.

Improved Longevity:
Some studies suggest that adherence to a vegan diet is associated with increased lifespan and a lower risk of premature mortality.

It's important to note that while a vegan diet offers many health benefits, it must be well-planned to ensure all essential nutrients are obtained. Consulting a registered dietitian or healthcare professional can provide guidance on creating a balanced and nutritionally adequate vegan meal plan tailored to individual needs and preferences.

Numerous studies and research findings support the health benefits of veganism. These studies have explored the impact of a vegan diet on various aspects of health, including cardiovascular health, weight management, diabetes prevention, and cancer risk reduction. Here are some key studies and research findings that highlight the health advantages of veganism:

The Adventist Health Study-2 (AHS-2): This long-term study of Seventh-day Adventists found that vegetarians and vegans had lower rates of heart disease, high blood pressure, and high cholesterol compared to non-vegetarians. The study suggested that a vegetarian diet, including veganism, is associated with a reduced risk of cardiovascular diseases.

EPIC-Oxford Study: This large-scale study found that vegetarians and vegans had a significantly lower risk of ischemic heart disease compared to meat-eaters. Vegans had the lowest risk among the groups studied.

The Adventist Mortality Study: Research involving Seventh-day Adventists found that vegetarians, including vegans, had a lower risk of developing type 2 diabetes compared to non-vegetarians.

The Diabetes Control and Complications Trial (DCCT): This study demonstrated that a low-fat, plant-based diet can effectively improve glycemic control in individuals with type 2 diabetes.

The AHS-2: The same study mentioned earlier found that vegans had the lowest average BMI among all dietary groups, suggesting that a vegan diet may be beneficial for weight management.

The EPIC-Oxford Study: Besides its findings on heart disease, this study also indicated that vegetarians, including vegans, had a lower overall cancer risk than meat-eaters. The risk reduction was particularly significant for certain types of cancer, such as colon and breast cancer.

The Dietary Approaches to Stop Hypertension (DASH) Diet: Research has shown that a plant-based diet, similar to veganism, aligns with the principles of the DASH diet, which is effective in lowering blood pressure.

A 2015 study published in the journal Frontiers in Nutrition found that a vegan diet rich in fruits, vegetables, and whole grains could help reduce symptoms in individuals with rheumatoid arthritis, possibly due to its anti-inflammatory properties.

A study published in the journal Nutrients in 2019 found that a vegan diet may be associated with a lower risk of developing inflammatory bowel disease (IBD) and may also be beneficial in managing symptoms in individuals with IBD.

The Blue Zones research, which examines areas with a high concentration of centenarians, has found that plant-based diets, including vegan diets, are common among populations with exceptional longevity.

These studies and research findings collectively suggest that a well-planned vegan diet can have significant health benefits, including reducing the risk of chronic diseases, improving cardiovascular health, and promoting overall well-being. However, it's crucial to emphasize that the quality and variety of foods within a vegan diet play a crucial role in achieving these health benefits. Consulting a registered dietitian can help individuals create a balanced and nutritionally adequate vegan meal plan tailored to their specific health goals.

Balanced vegan eating involves consuming a variety of plant-based foods to ensure you get all the essential nutrients your body needs for optimal health. Here's guidance on how to achieve a well-balanced vegan diet:

1. Emphasize Whole Plant Foods:

Base your meals on whole grains like brown rice, quinoa, and oats.
Include a variety of fruits and vegetables, aiming for different colors and types to maximize nutrient diversity.
Consume legumes like beans, lentils, and chickpeas as they are excellent sources of protein, fiber, and essential nutrients.

2. Include Protein-Rich Foods:
Incorporate protein sources such as tofu, tempeh, edamame, seitan, and plant-based meat substitutes if desired.
Nuts, seeds, and nut butters (e.g., almonds, chia seeds, and almond butter) also provide protein.

3. Don't Skip Healthy Fats:
Include sources of healthy fats like avocados, nuts, seeds, and olive oil in your diet. These fats are essential for overall health.
Consider adding ground flaxseeds or chia seeds to your meals for omega-3 fatty acids.

4. Ensure Adequate Calcium Intake:
Consume calcium-fortified plant-based milk, calcium-set tofu, leafy greens (e.g., kale, collard greens, and bok choy), and almonds to meet your calcium needs.

5. Meet Iron Requirements:

Include iron-rich foods such as legumes, tofu, quinoa, fortified cereals, and leafy greens.
Pair iron-rich foods with vitamin C-rich foods like citrus fruits, bell peppers, and strawberries to enhance iron absorption.

6. Prioritize Vitamin B12:

Consider taking a vitamin B12 supplement or consuming B12-fortified foods like plant-based milk, breakfast cereals, and nutritional yeast. Vitamin B12 is not naturally present in plant foods.

7. Include Iodine Sources:

Use iodized salt and consume iodine-fortified foods to ensure you meet your iodine needs. Seaweed can also be a source, but the iodine content can vary widely.

8. Optimize Vitamin D Intake:

Get regular sun exposure to help your body synthesize vitamin D. Depending on your location and sun exposure, you may need a vitamin D supplement.

9. Plan Balanced Meals:

Create balanced meals that include a source of protein, carbohydrates, healthy fats, and plenty of vegetables.
Experiment with various cooking methods and seasonings to enhance flavors and make your meals more enjoyable.

10. Stay Hydrated:

- Drink plenty of water throughout the day to maintain proper hydration.

11. Consider Supplements:

- Depending on individual needs and dietary choices, consider supplements like vitamin D, iodine, and omega-3 fatty acids, if required. Consult with a healthcare professional or registered dietitian for personalized recommendations.

12. Monitor Nutrient Intake:

- Periodically track your nutrient intake using a nutrition app or consult with a registered dietitian to ensure you're meeting your nutritional requirements.

Remember that balance and variety are key to a successful vegan diet. Experiment with different foods and recipes to keep your meals interesting and nutritious. A well-planned vegan diet can provide all the essential nutrients your body needs while promoting overall health and well-being.

Chapter 3: Making the Transition

I don't recommend going full vegan, from eating red meat, white meat, dairy, all at once. It is a big change for your body, and I would suggest starting slowly, as I did. Slow change is more stable, and makes it more likely that you will stick with it for the long term, and hopefully for the rest of your life.

One of the main struggles I've faced is being a vegan living among other carnivores. Make your intentions clear to your household what you are trying to accomplish, and let them know how they can support you. I found that letting my family know exactly what I can and cannot eat ahead of time, saved a lot of disappointment on both sides when family gatherings came around. Do not feel like you are being picky or difficult, your health should be your number one priority and if your family cares about you, which I am sure they do, they will support you and make you a meat/dairy free serving at dinner.

If you are starting to wean yourself off from red meat, buy a salmon filet or chicken breast to cook for dinner. Ground turkey is a good substitute for ground beef, and you can make turkey tacos or burgers, and you will notice there is a lot less fat and oil.

Go buy a small "food journal" and record your meal plan, what you actually eat, and then HOW YOU FEEL AFTER EATING. This is especially important in training yourself, by reinforcing the good feelings you get when eating healthy, so, document it! Instagram your meals as well, some may find it annoying, but it is a great way to make yourself accountable and share with the world your healthy choices to inspire others. Even when you slip up and make a mistake, say, finishing your child's half eaten hot dog, record it in your journal. Record any bad feelings you feel afterwards. This is not a shaming activity but a learning activity. By recording that you felt indigestion, or fatigue after finishing your child's hot dog, you will be more likely to remember those feelings in the future and not make the same mistake again. I always feel bad wasting food, so when my kids don't finish their food, and it's something I cannot eat myself, I let my dog have it. Win-win situation.

Once you are ready to eliminate poultry, I would suggest keeping eggs and fish in your diet, and make sure to eat plenty of vegetables rather than grains and starches. I started taking a multivitamin and B12 supplement as insurance, so I can make sure I don't miss out on any nutrients by cutting out all of the meat. It is important to be vigilant about the source of your eggs and fish. Most farm-raised salmon are known to carry disease and with lake salmon you run the risk of mercury, so try limiting your fish meals to 2-3 servings per week. All the more reason to eliminate fish next!

It may seem intimidating to jump right into being a vegan, but if you slowly move towards this lifestyle, eliminating dairy will seem like the logical next step. Within weeks of eliminating dairy I noticed that my skin was remarkably clearer, and my energy levels were higher than ever. There were a few times when I would finish my kids ice cream, and I would notice how tired and gross I would feel afterwards, that I realized there was no going back to dairy, ever again. Don't be discouraged, because there probably will be times where you have no other choices and will have to eat dairy, but make sure you document how you feel afterwards, and let your heart be your guide.

Overcoming common psychological barriers to becoming vegan can be a challenging but rewarding process. Here are some strategies to help individuals address these barriers and make a successful transition to a vegan lifestyle.

Educate Yourself:
Learn about the ethical, environmental, and health reasons for choosing a vegan lifestyle. Understanding the impact of your choices can provide motivation and a sense of purpose.

Set Realistic Goals:
Start by setting achievable, short-term goals. For example, you can commit to eating one vegan meal per day or participating in "Meatless Mondays" before transitioning fully.

Find a Support System:
Connect with like-minded individuals, whether through vegan social groups, online communities, or local meetups. Support from others who share your values can be invaluable.

Plan Your Transition:
Gradual transitions may be less overwhelming. Create a plan that includes a timeline for reducing or eliminating animal products from your diet and lifestyle.

Experiment with New Foods:
Explore the variety of vegan foods available. Trying new recipes and cuisines can make the transition more enjoyable and reduce feelings of deprivation.

Seek Nutritional Guidance:
Concerns about nutrient adequacy are common. Consult with a registered dietitian or nutritionist who specializes in plant-based diets to ensure you are meeting your nutritional needs.

Mindfulness and Coping Strategies:

Recognize and address any emotional or psychological challenges that arise during the transition. Mindfulness practices, stress management techniques, and seeking professional support when needed can be helpful.

Address Social Pressure:
Be prepared for questions and criticism from friends and family. Educate them about your choices and the reasons behind them, but also be patient and understanding of their perspectives.

Meal Planning and Preparation:
Invest time in meal planning and preparation to ensure you have satisfying and convenient vegan options readily available. This can prevent relying on non-vegan choices out of convenience.

Explore Vegan Alternatives:
Discover vegan alternatives to your favorite non-vegan foods, such as plant-based milk, vegan cheese, and meat substitutes. Many of these products closely mimic the taste and texture of animal-derived equivalents.

Celebrate Milestones:
Acknowledge and celebrate your achievements along the way. Each step you take toward a vegan lifestyle is a significant accomplishment.

Keep up with the latest information, recipes, and resources related to veganism. This can keep your enthusiasm high and help you stay committed. Understand that transitioning to a vegan lifestyle is a process, and it's okay to make mistakes along the way. Every effort you make counts toward a more compassionate and sustainable lifestyle. Periodically revisit the reasons you decided to become vegan. Remind yourself of your ethical, environmental, and health motivations to stay committed.

Consider sharing your experiences and knowledge with others. Advocating for veganism and helping others understand your perspective can be rewarding and reinforce your commitment.

Overcoming psychological barriers to becoming vegan may take time and effort, but with determination and support, many people successfully make the transition and find it to be a fulfilling and positive lifestyle choice.

Transitioning to veganism, whether gradually or immediately, has its pros and cons, and the choice depends on individual preferences, circumstances, and motivations. Here's a breakdown of the advantages and disadvantages of each approach:

Transitioning Gradually:

Pros:

Gradual transitions can feel less overwhelming and reduce the fear of giving up favorite foods all at once.

 You have time to learn about vegan nutrition, discover new recipes, and explore plant-based options without rushing.

 For some, gradual changes are more sustainable in the long term, allowing time to adjust to new habits and preferences.

It may be easier to adapt socially, as you can still participate in non-vegan meals with friends and family while gradually incorporating vegan options.

Slowly increasing fiber intake can help your digestive system adjust to a higher-fiber diet, potentially reducing discomfort.

Cons:

It may take longer to fully align with your ethical, environmental, or health goals.

Some individuals might get stuck in a semi-vegetarian phase, never fully embracing a vegan lifestyle.

Transitioning Immediately (Cold Turkey):

Pros:

You immediately reduce harm to animals and your environmental footprint.

It sends a clear signal to yourself and others about your commitment to veganism.

Once you decide to go vegan, there's no need to constantly make choices about which foods to exclude or include.

Some health benefits, such as reduced cholesterol levels, may be seen more quickly.

Cons:

The abrupt change can be emotionally challenging, leading to cravings or feelings of deprivation.

You might feel pressure to quickly learn about vegan nutrition and find suitable alternatives.

Immediate transitions can be more challenging in social situations, such as dining out with non-vegan friends or family.

 A sudden increase in fiber can lead to digestive discomfort for some individuals.

In some cases, the abrupt change may lead to relapses if cravings become overwhelming.

Ultimately, the best approach varies from person to person. Some people thrive on immediate transitions, while others find gradual changes more sustainable. Consider your personality, motivations, support system, and resources when deciding which approach suits you best. Additionally, seeking guidance from a registered dietitian or vegan support groups can be valuable regardless of the transition method you choose.

Reading food labels to identify animal-derived ingredients can be a helpful skill for vegans and individuals with dietary restrictions. Here are some tips on how to read food labels effectively:

- Look for allergen labels or statements that explicitly list common allergens like milk, eggs, fish, shellfish, tree nuts, peanuts, wheat, and soy. If you see one of these allergens listed, it's a clear indication that the product contains animal-derived ingredients.
- Be familiar with common animal-derived ingredients like milk, lactose, casein, whey, eggs, gelatin, and certain colorings like carmine (cochineal) and natural red 4 (also known as E120).
- The ingredient list on food labels is your most valuable resource. Ingredients are typically listed in descending order of quantity, meaning the ingredient that appears first is the most abundant. Look for animal-derived ingredients throughout the list.

Watch for Hidden Animal Products. Some animal-derived ingredients may have less obvious names. For example, rennet, a common cheese-making enzyme, is of animal origin. Gelatin may be listed simply as "gelatin" or under its E number (E441).

Be Wary of Common Food Additives, some food additives, such as certain colorings, flavorings, and emulsifiers, may be derived from animals. Research and familiarize yourself with these additives.

Look for Vegan-Certified Labels. Some products carry vegan-certified labels or logos, making it easy to identify vegan-friendly options. These labels indicate that the product does not contain animal-derived ingredients. If you're unsure about the ingredients in a specific product, consider reaching out to the manufacturer. They can provide information about the sourcing and origin of ingredients. There are smartphone apps available that can scan barcodes and provide information about whether a product is vegan or not. Examples include "Is It Vegan?" and "Bunny Free." Stay updated on food labeling regulations and changes in ingredient names. Manufacturers may reformulate products or change ingredient sources over time.

Read Both Product and Packaging Label - Ingredients might be listed on the product itself as well as on the outer packaging. Be sure to check both if you're uncertain. Remember that labeling practices can vary by region and country, so it's important to familiarize yourself with the specific labeling conventions in your area. Additionally, if you have specific dietary concerns or allergies, consult with a healthcare professional or registered dietitian for personalized guidance on reading food labels.

Meal planning is a critical element of starting your Vegan Transition, and cooking as a vegan can be enjoyable and fulfilling with a bit of preparation and creativity. Here are some meal planning and cooking tips for vegans:

Start with achievable meal planning goals, such as planning for a few days or a week at a time.Plan your meals for the week ahead, including breakfast, lunch, dinner, and snacks. Having a menu can reduce decision-making stress.Ensure your meals include a balance of protein, carbohydrates, healthy fats, and a variety of colorful vegetables and fruits. Make a shopping list based on your menu plan and stick to it to minimize impulse purchases. Shopping with a list can also save you time.Prepare larger quantities of staples like grains, legumes, and sauces to use throughout the week. This can save you time on busy days.Embrace variety by trying new grains (e.g., quinoa, farro), legumes (e.g., lentils, chickpeas), vegetables, and plant-based proteins. Experiment with herbs and spices to add flavor and variety to your dishes. Options like basil, cumin, turmeric, and garlic can transform a simple meal.

Familiarize yourself with different cooking techniques, including sautéing, roasting, steaming, and stir-frying, to create diverse and delicious vegan meals.Create your own salad dressings, pasta sauces, and marinades using plant-based ingredients like olive oil, vinegar, tahini, and soy sauce. Explore meat substitutes like tempeh, tofu, seitan, and plant-based burger patties. These can add variety and texture to your meals.Ensure you get enough protein from sources like legumes, tofu, tempeh, and plant-based protein powders if needed. Try different plant-based milk options like almond, soy, oat, and coconut milk for cooking and baking.

Many baked goods can be made vegan by substituting eggs with flaxseeds or applesauce, and dairy with plant-based milk and butter. Create colorful salads and Buddha bowls with a mix of grains, greens, roasted vegetables, nuts, seeds, and a tasty dressing. Nutritional yeast adds a cheesy, savory flavor to dishes. Sprinkle it on pasta, popcorn, or use it in sauces and vegan cheese recipes. Keep simple, quick-to-prepare ingredients on hand for busy days. This might include canned beans, pre-washed greens, and frozen vegetables. Cook larger portions and use leftovers for the next day's lunch or dinner. This can save time and reduce food waste.Properly store and handle plant-based ingredients to prevent contamination and foodborne illness. Cooking can be a creative and joyful process. Enjoy the experience, and don't be afraid to experiment with flavors and ingredients. Explore vegan cookbooks, websites, and cooking videos for inspiration and new recipes. Social Media sites such as TikTok and Pinterest are loaded with vegan content and communities.

Remember that cooking as a vegan can be an exciting journey of discovery. Don't be discouraged if a dish doesn't turn out perfectly the first time; practice makes perfect. As you become more comfortable with vegan cooking, you'll develop your own favorite recipes and techniques.

Once you have mastered the careful planning for your Vegan transition, you will also have to plan on how to respond to criticism and questions from your friends and family on your new lifestyle with grace. It is important to maintain positive relationships and promote understanding, not just for the Vegan Community but for your own mental health. Here are some tips on how to do so:

Approach conversations with a calm and patient demeanor. Remember that people may not fully understand your choice, and it might take time for them to come to terms with it. When someone criticizes or questions your choice, listen attentively to their concerns or comments. Show that you value their perspective and are open to discussion.
Avoid becoming defensive or confrontational. Instead, respond in a non-confrontational and respectful manner. If someone has misconceptions about veganism, gently and politely share accurate information about your reasons for choosing a vegan lifestyle. Use evidence-based facts to support your arguments. You can also share your personal experiences and the positive impacts of going vegan on your health, the environment, or animal welfare. Personal stories can be compelling. Express your feelings and choices using "I" statements. For example, say, "I chose to go vegan because I believe it aligns with my values," rather than making absolute statements like, "Veganism is the only right way." Provide resources like books, documentaries, or websites that have helped you learn more about veganism. This allows others to explore the topic at their own pace.

Just as you expect respect for your choices, respect the dietary choices of others. Avoid judgment or criticism of their dietary preferences. Not every criticism or question requires a lengthy response. Sometimes, a simple acknowledgment of the comment and a polite change of subject can be more effective. Highlight shared values or concerns. If someone expresses concern about animal welfare, for instance, you can discuss your shared compassion for animals. Show that being vegan doesn't mean missing out on delicious and satisfying meals. Share vegan dishes with family and friends to demonstrate that vegan food can be enjoyable. Changing perspectives may take time. Continue to live your vegan lifestyle with conviction, and over time, you may influence others positively. Sometimes, despite your best efforts, others may not fully understand or accept your choice. In such cases, it's okay to agree to disagree and maintain respectful boundaries.

Connect with vegan communities or support groups to share experiences and find advice on how to handle criticism and questions from loved ones. Remember that your choice to go vegan is a personal one, and while you can share your reasons and educate others, you cannot control their responses or choices. Approach these conversations with empathy and the intent to foster understanding, and over time, you may find that your loved ones become more accepting and supportive of your decision.

Plant Based Meat Alternatives

Plant-based alternatives for meat, dairy, and eggs have become increasingly popular and widely available. These alternatives offer a cruelty-free and sustainable way to enjoy familiar tastes and textures. Tofu is a versatile soy-based protein that comes in various textures (silken, soft, firm, extra-firm) and can be used in a wide range of savory and sweet dishes. Tempeh is a fermented soybean product that has a nutty flavor and firm texture. It's great for grilling, stir-frying, or crumbling into dishes. Seitan, also known as wheat gluten, has a chewy texture similar to meat. It's a protein-rich option often used in vegan "meat" dishes. Textured Vegetable Protein (TVP) is made from soy flour and is a common meat substitute. It's often used in dishes like chili, tacos, and spaghetti sauce.

There are various brands of vegan burger patties available, made from ingredients like mushrooms, beans, soy, or vegetables. Vegan sausages made from ingredients like seitan, lentils, or vegetables offer a meaty texture and flavor. Young, unripe jackfruit has a mild flavor and shreds like pulled pork. It's often used in barbecue or curry dishes.
Portobello, shiitake, and oyster mushrooms can be grilled, roasted, or sautéed to create a meaty texture and umami flavor.

Plant-Based Milk options include almond milk, soy milk, oat milk, coconut milk, and rice milk. These are used as substitutes for cow's milk in recipes and beverages. There are dairy-free yogurt alternatives made from soy, almond, coconut, and cashews, available in various flavors. Plant-based cheeses are made from nuts (cashews, almonds), soy, or coconut and come in various forms, including slices, shreds, and spreads. Butter made from plant oils like coconut, avocado, or olive oil is used for spreading, baking, and cooking. Coconut cream or cashew cream can be used in recipes that call for heavy cream.

Crumbled tofu, seasoned with spices and vegetables, makes a great substitute for scrambled eggs. Chickpea flour, when mixed with water and spices, can be used to make vegan omelets or quiches. There are various commercial egg replacers on the market that work well in baking and cooking. Ground flax or chia seeds mixed with water can be used as an egg substitute in recipes that require binding. Silken tofu can be blended into smoothies and used in baking to add moisture and binding.

These plant-based alternatives provide options for vegans and those looking to reduce their consumption of animal products. The choice of which alternative to use depends on personal preferences and the specific dish you're preparing. Experimenting with different options can help you discover your favorite plant-based substitutes for meat, dairy, and eggs.

Building Your Vegan Pantry

Building a well-stocked vegan pantry involves having a variety of essential ingredients on hand to make cooking and meal preparation easier. Here's a list of key ingredients to consider:

1. Grains:
Brown rice
Quinoa
Whole wheat pasta
Rolled oats
Barley
Bulgur

2. Legumes:
Canned or dried beans (black, kidney, chickpeas, lentils, etc.)
Split peas
Red or green lentils

3. Canned and Jarred Goods:
Canned tomatoes (diced, crushed, and tomato sauce)
Tomato paste
Vegetable broth or bouillon cubes
Coconut milk
Nut butters (peanut, almond, etc.)
Tahini (sesame seed paste)
Pickles, olives, and capers

4. Nuts and Seeds:
Almonds
Walnuts
Cashews
Chia seeds
Flaxseeds
Sunflower seeds
Pumpkin seeds

5. Plant-Based Protein:
Tofu (silken, firm, extra-firm)
Tempeh
Seitan

Textured vegetable protein (TVP)

6. Non-Dairy Milk:
Almond milk
Soy milk
Oat milk
Coconut milk (canned and carton)
Rice milk

7. Condiments and Sauces:
Soy sauce or tamari (for a gluten-free option)
Vegan Worcestershire sauce
Mustard (Dijon, yellow)
Ketchup
Sriracha or hot sauce
Vegan mayonnaise
Nutritional yeast (for a cheesy flavor)
Vegan salad dressings

8. Herbs and Spices:
Basil
Oregano
Thyme
Rosemary
Cumin
Paprika
Chili powder
Turmeric
Garlic powder
Onion powder
Salt and black pepper

9. Baking Supplies:
All-purpose flour (or alternative flours like almond or coconut)
Baking powder
Baking soda
Agave nectar or maple syrup (as sweeteners)
Vegan chocolate chips or cocoa powder

10. Cooking Oils:

- Olive oil
- Coconut oil
- Vegetable oil

11. Pasta and Rice:
- Various pasta shapes (spaghetti, penne, macaroni)
- White and brown rice
- Risotto rice (e.g., Arborio)

12. Flour and Starches:
- Cornstarch (used for thickening sauces)
- Whole wheat or gluten-free flour

13. Dried Herbs and Spices:
- Parsley
- Sage
- Bay leaves
- Cinnamon
- Nutmeg

14. Sweeteners:
- Sugar (white and brown)
- Maple syrup
- Agave nectar

15. Vinegars:
- White vinegar
- Apple cider vinegar
- Balsamic vinegar

16. Asian Ingredients:
- Rice vinegar
- Sesame oil
- Tamari or soy sauce

17. Canned Vegetables and Fruits:
- Canned corn
- Canned peas
- Canned pineapple
- Canned diced tomatoes

18. Vegan Snacks:
- Popcorn kernels
- Vegan crackers
- Rice cakes

19. Vegan Soup and Bouillon Bases:
- Vegan vegetable broth or bouillon cubes
- Miso paste

20. Ethnic Ingredients:
- Curry paste
- Coconut cream
- Garam masala
- Tofu noodles (for Asian dishes)

Having these essential ingredients in your vegan pantry can serve as a foundation for creating a wide range of delicious and nutritious vegan meals. As you become more comfortable with vegan cooking, you can expand your pantry with additional items tailored to your preferences and the types of dishes you enjoy making.

Creating DIY vegan versions of common ingredients allows you to have control over the ingredients used and often results in cost-effective and customized options. Here are some DIY vegan versions of common ingredients:

Vegan Butter:
Ingredients: Coconut oil, refined coconut oil (for stability), non-dairy milk, salt, and a bit of turmeric for color.
Instructions: Melt the coconut oil, blend it with the other ingredients, and let it solidify in the fridge.

Vegan Mayonnaise:

Ingredients: Silken tofu, lemon juice, vinegar, mustard, sugar, salt, and oil (optional).
Instructions: Blend all the ingredients until smooth, adding oil for creaminess if desired.

Nut Milk:
Ingredients: Nuts (e.g., almonds, cashews), water, and sweetener or flavorings (optional).
Instructions: Soak the nuts, blend them with water, and strain through a nut milk bag or cheesecloth.

Vegan Sour Cream:
Ingredients: Cashews, lemon juice, vinegar, water, and salt.
Instructions: Blend all ingredients until smooth, adjusting water for desired consistency.

Vegan Cheese:
Ingredients: Cashews, nutritional yeast, lemon juice, garlic, salt, and water.
Instructions: Blend all ingredients until creamy, adding water as needed.

Vegan Cream Cheese:
Ingredients: Cashews, lemon juice, vinegar, nutritional yeast, garlic, salt, and water.
Instructions: Blend ingredients until creamy, adding water as needed.

Vegan Ricotta Cheese:
Ingredients: Tofu, lemon juice, nutritional yeast, garlic, salt, and olive oil (optional).
Instructions: Blend ingredients until it resembles the texture of ricotta cheese.

Vegan Parmesan Cheese:
Ingredients: Cashews, nutritional yeast, garlic powder, and salt.
Instructions: Blend all ingredients until they resemble grated Parmesan cheese.

Vegan Egg Substitute:
Ingredients: Flaxseeds or chia seeds and water.
Instructions: Mix one tablespoon of ground flaxseeds or chia seeds with three tablespoons of water and let it sit until it thickens (acts as an egg binder in recipes).

Homemade Vegan Bread:
- Ingredients: Flour, yeast, water, sugar, salt, and optional plant-based milk or oil.
- Instructions: Mix and knead the ingredients, let the dough rise, then bake.

Vegan BBQ Sauce:
- Ingredients: Tomato sauce, molasses, vinegar, sugar, spices, and soy sauce.
- Instructions: Mix all ingredients in a saucepan and simmer until thickened.

Vegan Pesto:
- Ingredients: Basil, pine nuts, garlic, nutritional yeast, olive oil, and lemon juice.
- Instructions: Blend all ingredients until smooth.

These DIY vegan versions of common ingredients can be customized to your taste preferences and dietary needs. They're also a great way to experiment with flavors and textures, making your vegan meals more enjoyable and satisfying.

Tools for Cooking Vegan Meals

Cooking vegan meals doesn't require any specialized tools, but having the right kitchen equipment can make your cooking experience more efficient and enjoyable. Here are some must-have tools for cooking vegan meals:

- A sharp, reliable chef's knife is essential for chopping, slicing, and dicing vegetables, fruits, and other ingredients.
- Invest in a sturdy, easy-to-clean cutting board to protect your countertops and provide a safe cutting surface.
- Blender or Food Processor: These appliances are versatile for making smoothies, soups, sauces, vegan cheeses, and creamy dips.
- Immersion Blender: Handy for blending soups and sauces directly in the pot without transferring them to a countertop blender.
- A good-quality skillet or pan is essential for sautéing, frying, and cooking a wide range of vegan dishes.
- Various-sized pots are useful for boiling pasta, cooking grains, simmering soups, and preparing stews.
- Baking sheets are handy for roasting vegetables, while pans are essential for baking vegan desserts and casseroles.
- A steamer basket allows you to cook vegetables, grains, and dumplings without losing their nutrients and flavors.
- Colander or Strainer: Essential for draining cooked pasta, beans, and vegetables.
- Tofu Press: - If you use tofu frequently, a tofu press helps remove excess moisture, making it easier to marinate and cook.
- Grater and Zester: - Useful for grating vegetables, fruits, and vegan cheeses, as well as zesting citrus fruits.
- Measuring Cups and Spoons: - Accurate measurements are crucial for successful vegan baking and cooking.
- Mixing Bowls: - A variety of mixing bowls in different sizes allows you to prepare and store ingredients easily.
- Whisk: - For mixing and aerating wet ingredients, sauces, and dressings.
- Wooden Spatula and Silicone Spatula: - These utensils are gentle on cookware and perfect for stirring, flipping, and scraping.
- Microplane: - Great for finely grating spices, garlic, ginger, and citrus zest.
- Can Opener: - For opening cans of beans, tomatoes, and other canned ingredients.
- Vegetable Peeler: - Useful for peeling vegetables and fruits or creating thin strips of vegetables for salads and dishes.

- Food Storage Containers: - Have a variety of airtight containers for storing leftovers, prepped ingredients, and packed lunches.
- Instant-Read Thermometer: - Ensures that your vegan proteins (e.g., tofu, tempeh) are cooked to the right temperature for safe consumption.
- Spiralizer: - Great for creating vegetable noodles (zoodles) and adding variety to your dishes.

These kitchen tools are versatile and will help you prepare a wide range of vegan meals efficiently. As you gain experience in vegan cooking, you may discover additional tools that suit your specific cooking style and preferences.

Simple Recipes for Beginners

If you're new to vegan cooking, starting with simple and delicious recipes can make your transition to a vegan lifestyle easier and more enjoyable. Here are some beginner-friendly vegan recipes:

Vegan Pasta Primavera:
Cook your favorite pasta, toss it with sautéed seasonal vegetables (such as bell peppers, zucchini, and cherry tomatoes), and drizzle with a homemade vegan pesto or marinara sauce. Top with fresh basil and nutritional yeast or vegan Parmesan for added flavor.

Vegan Chickpea Salad Sandwich:
Mash canned chickpeas with a fork and mix them with vegan mayo, diced celery, red onion, pickle relish, and your choice of seasonings (like garlic powder and paprika). Spread it on whole-grain bread with lettuce and tomato.

Vegan Stir-Fry:
Stir-fry your favorite vegetables (such as bell peppers, broccoli, and snap peas) with tofu or tempeh in a soy sauce-based sauce. Serve over cooked rice or noodles.

Vegan Chili:
Sauté onions, garlic, and bell peppers in a large pot. Add canned beans (kidney, black, and pinto), canned diced tomatoes, chili powder, cumin, and paprika. Simmer until flavors meld together. Top with chopped green onions and vegan sour cream.

Vegan Quinoa Bowl:
Cook quinoa and serve it in a bowl with a variety of toppings like sautéed kale, roasted sweet potatoes, avocado slices, and a tahini dressing.

Vegan Lentil Soup:
Sauté onions, carrots, and celery in a pot. Add dried green or brown lentils, vegetable broth, canned diced tomatoes, and your favorite spices (like cumin and thyme). Simmer until the lentils are tender.

Vegan Oatmeal:
Cook oats with non-dairy milk (like almond milk), sweeten with maple syrup or agave nectar, and top with fresh fruit, nuts, and a sprinkle of cinnamon.

Vegan Tacos:

Fill soft or hard taco shells with seasoned black beans, sautéed onions and peppers, salsa, guacamole, and shredded lettuce. You can also add vegan cheese or cashew cream.

Vegan Buddha Bowl:

Combine cooked quinoa or brown rice with roasted or steamed vegetables, baked tofu or tempeh, and a drizzle of tahini or peanut sauce. Garnish with sesame seeds and chopped fresh herbs.

Vegan Smoothie:

Blend frozen mixed berries, a banana, spinach or kale, almond milk, and a spoonful of peanut butter for a nutritious and tasty breakfast or snack.

Vegan Avocado Toast:

Spread ripe avocado on whole-grain toast and top with sliced tomatoes, red pepper flakes, salt, and a squeeze of lemon juice.

Vegan Baked Potatoes:

Bake potatoes until tender, then top with vegan butter, sautéed mushrooms, spinach, and vegan cheese. Bake until the cheese melts.

These beginner-friendly vegan recipes are easy to prepare and can be customized with your favorite ingredients and flavors. As you become more comfortable with vegan cooking, you can explore more complex recipes and expand your plant-based culinary skills.

Eating Out

Communicating your vegan dietary needs to waitstaff at a restaurant is an important step in ensuring that you receive a vegan meal that aligns with your preferences and requirements. To effectively communicate your dietary needs to waitstaff, be Clear and Specific. Use clear and simple language to convey that you are vegan. You can say, "I am vegan," or "I follow a vegan diet." Politely ask questions about the menu items to ensure they meet your vegan criteria. For example, you can ask if a dish contains any animal products, such as meat, dairy, eggs, or honey. Let the waitstaff know if you have any specific dietary preferences or restrictions beyond being vegan. For instance, if you're avoiding gluten or nuts, mention this as well. If a menu item can be made vegan with minor modifications, kindly ask if they can accommodate your request. For example, you can ask for a dish without cheese or with tofu instead of meat.
Be Polite and Patient: Approach the conversation with a polite and patient attitude. Remember that some wait staff may not be familiar with veganism, so be prepared to explain your needs. If you're unsure about certain ingredients, ask if they can provide a list or check with the kitchen staff for a complete ingredient breakdown. Show appreciation for their assistance and understanding. Thank them for helping you find vegan options or for making accommodations.

If you have dietary restrictions beyond veganism, you can use restaurant apps or websites that provide dietary information and options. Some apps even allow you to communicate your dietary needs directly to the restaurant.

Once you've communicated your needs and placed your order, it's a good practice to double-check with the waitstaff or manager when your meal is served to ensure it meets your dietary requirements. Remember that most restaurants are willing to accommodate dietary needs, including veganism, as long as they are informed in advance. By communicating your needs clearly and respectfully, you can enjoy a satisfying vegan dining experience while helping raise awareness about vegan options in restaurants.

Traveling

Finding vegan options on the road can be a bit challenging, especially in areas where vegan-friendly restaurants are less common. However, with some strategies and planning, you can enjoy vegan meals while traveling. Before your trip, research vegan-friendly restaurants, cafes, and grocery stores at your destination. Websites and apps like HappyCow, Yelp, and Google Maps can be invaluable for finding vegan options.

If you're taking a road trip, plan your stops in advance to include cities or towns known for their vegan food scene. This way, you can ensure you have access to vegan options along the way. Carry a variety of vegan snacks like trail mix, energy bars, fresh fruit, and cut-up veggies. These snacks can keep you satisfied between meals. Download and use vegan-specific apps like HappyCow, Vegman, or Vanilla Bean to locate vegan-friendly eateries near your location. If you find a restaurant that looks promising but doesn't have clearly marked vegan options on the menu, call ahead and ask if they can accommodate your dietary needs. If you have access to a cooler, bring perishable vegan items like vegan cheese, hummus, and pre-made salads to have on hand during your journey.

Don't be afraid to customize your order at non-vegan restaurants. Many places are willing to make substitutions or modifications to existing menu items to make them vegan. Restaurants serving international cuisines like Thai, Indian, Mexican, and Mediterranean often have vegan options or dishes that can easily be made vegan.

Visit local grocery stores or supermarkets to pick up vegan staples like fresh produce, nuts, seeds, bread, and non-dairy milk. You can create simple meals with these ingredients.
Ask Locals for Recommendations:

Don't hesitate to ask locals for their recommendations on vegan-friendly places to eat. They may be aware of hidden gems that may not appear in online searches. If you're staying in a hotel, inquire about vegan breakfast options or if they can accommodate vegan requests. Look for accommodations that cater to vegans or have vegan-friendly options available in their restaurants or breakfast menus.

If traveling internationally, learn some basic vegan phrases in the local language to communicate your dietary needs more effectively.

Be prepared to be flexible and creative with your meals, especially in areas with limited vegan options. You can often create a satisfying meal from sides or appetizers.

After your trip, consider leaving reviews on restaurant review websites or apps to help other travelers find vegan options in the same locations. By combining these strategies and planning ahead, you can navigate your road trip or travel adventure as a vegan, ensuring you have access to delicious and satisfying plant-based meals along the way.

Chapter 4: Long Term Nutritional Considerations

Going vegan can have numerous health benefits, but it's essential to pay attention to long-term nutritional considerations to ensure you maintain a well-balanced and healthy diet. Protein is essential for overall health. Ensure you get an adequate amount of protein from plant-based sources like beans, lentils, tofu, tempeh, quinoa, nuts, seeds, and plant-based protein supplements if needed. Vitamin B12 is not naturally found in plant foods, so it's crucial for vegans to obtain it from fortified foods (such as plant-based milk, nutritional yeast, and breakfast cereals) or B12 supplements. Plant-based iron sources include legumes, fortified cereals, whole grains, nuts, seeds, and leafy greens. Consuming vitamin C-rich foods alongside iron-rich foods can enhance iron absorption.

To meet calcium needs, consume calcium-fortified plant milk, tofu made with calcium sulfate, leafy greens, almonds, and tahini. Vitamin D can be challenging to obtain from food alone, so consider getting adequate sun exposure (when possible) or taking a vitamin D supplement. Some plant-based milk and cereals are also fortified with vitamin D. Include sources of alpha-linolenic acid (ALA), such as flaxseeds, chia seeds, hemp seeds, and walnuts, in your diet. Consider an algae-based omega-3 supplement for long-term health. Vegan diets may be lower in iodine, so include iodized salt in your diet or consume foods like seaweed (in moderation) and iodine-fortified products. Plant-based sources of zinc include legumes, whole grains, nuts, seeds, and fortified cereals. Ensure you have a varied diet to meet zinc needs.

Vegan diets are typically high in fiber, which is beneficial for digestive health. Ensure you drink plenty of water to prevent digestive discomfort. Consider regular blood tests and consult a healthcare provider or registered dietitian to determine if you need specific nutrient supplements. Consume a variety of plant foods to ensure you get a wide range of nutrients. Eating a rainbow of fruits and vegetables is a good guideline.

Plan your meals thoughtfully to ensure that you're meeting your nutritional needs. Include a balance of grains, legumes, vegetables, fruits, nuts, and seeds. Pay attention to bone health by consuming calcium-rich foods and engaging in weight training exercise to support bone density. Stay well-hydrated by drinking water throughout the day, as it is essential for overall health. Schedule regular check-ups with a healthcare provider to monitor your overall health and address any nutritional concerns. Continue to educate yourself about vegan nutrition, as research and guidelines may evolve over time.

Remember that everyone's nutritional needs are unique, and individual factors like age, gender, activity level, and health conditions can influence dietary requirements. It's advisable to consult with a registered dietitian or healthcare provider to create a personalized vegan nutrition plan that ensures you meet all your long-term nutritional needs.

Chapter 5: Beyond the Vegan Diet

Expanding beyond diet to embrace other aspects of vegan living involves adopting a more holistic approach that aligns with the ethical, environmental, and sustainable principles of veganism. Here are ways to incorporate veganism into various aspects of your life beyond just your diet:

Choose clothing and accessories made from synthetic, plant-based, or sustainable materials rather than animal-derived materials like leather, wool, and silk. Look for cruelty-free and vegan-certified brands. Opt for cruelty-free and vegan cosmetics, skincare, and personal care products. Many companies now offer vegan alternatives and avoid animal testing. Select cleaning and household products that are cruelty-free and eco-friendly. Avoid those that contain animal-derived ingredients or have been tested on animals.

Avoid activities that exploit animals for entertainment, such as circuses with animals, horse racing, and marine parks with captive dolphins and whales. If you're considering adopting a pet, choose a rescue animal from a shelter or rescue organization instead of supporting the breeding industry. Make sure to provide a loving and vegan-friendly home for your pet.

Consider ethical investing by supporting companies and investments that align with your vegan values, such as those involved in sustainable agriculture, clean energy, or cruelty-free products. Get involved in animal rights and vegan advocacy efforts. Join local or online vegan groups, participate in protests, and use your voice to raise awareness about animal welfare issues. Support vegan-friendly businesses, restaurants, and products to encourage the growth of the vegan economy. Continuously educate yourself about animal rights, environmental issues, and the health benefits of a vegan lifestyle. Share this information with others to inspire change.

Engage in open and respectful conversations with friends and family about your vegan choices. Encourage them to try vegan meals and respect your values. Connect with like-minded individuals in your community or online to share experiences and support each other on your vegan journey. When traveling, research vegan-friendly destinations, accommodations, and restaurants. Be prepared with vegan snacks for long journeys. Stay informed about policy changes and support legislation that promotes animal welfare and environmental sustainability. Be a role model by living compassionately and sustainably. Your actions and choices can inspire others to make more ethical and eco-conscious decisions.

Remember that transitioning to a fully vegan lifestyle doesn't happen overnight. It's a journey, and you can take gradual steps to incorporate these aspects into your life. The key is to align your values with your actions and make choices that reflect your commitment to a compassionate and sustainable way of living.

Promoting Veganism and Animal Rights

Getting involved in promoting veganism and animal rights can be a meaningful and impactful way to advocate for the well-being of animals and the adoption of a cruelty-free lifestyle. Look for local or national animal welfare organizations that align with your values and offer volunteer opportunities. You can help with animal care, fundraising, events, and advocacy efforts. Volunteer your time or donate to animal sanctuaries and rescue organizations that provide shelter and care for rescued animals. Attend vegan festivals, conferences, and expos to connect with like-minded individuals, learn from experts, and discover new vegan products and initiatives. Participate in or create local vegan meetup groups to build a community of like-minded individuals who can share resources, organize events, and support each other.

Use social media platforms to share information, articles, and resources related to veganism and animal rights. Engage in respectful discussions to raise awareness. Start a blog, vlog, or podcast focused on veganism, animal rights, and sustainable living. Share your experiences, recipes, and knowledge to educate and inspire others. Advocate for animal-friendly policies and legislation by contacting your local and national representatives, signing petitions, and participating in campaigns organized by animal rights organizations. Hand out vegan literature and engage in conversations with the public at events, fairs, and on college campuses. Tabling at local markets or community events can also be effective. Plan and host vegan outreach events, such as cooking demonstrations, film screenings, panel discussions, and guest speaker talks, to inform and engage your community.

Organize fundraisers or charity events to support animal welfare organizations. This can include bake sales, charity runs, or donation drives. Support Vegan Brands and Products: - Choose to support vegan brands and products that prioritize animal welfare and ethical practices. Promote these products to your network. Collaborate with local businesses, restaurants, and community centers to host vegan events or workshops. Engage in open and respectful conversations with friends and family about veganism. Share information and resources to help them better understand the lifestyle. Connect with other vegan activists, locally and online, to exchange ideas, share resources, and work on joint campaigns and initiatives. Stay informed about and advocate for animal rights legislation in your area. Attend town hall meetings and public hearings to voice your support for animal-friendly policies. If you're passionate about animal rights, consider pursuing a career in this field, whether as an animal rights lawyer, activist, researcher, or educator.

Remember that advocacy efforts can take various forms, and there's no one-size-fits-all approach. Find the methods that resonate most with you and align with your strengths and interests. Every effort counts in raising awareness about veganism and animal rights and creating a more compassionate world for animals.

Inspiring Others to Switch to Veganism

Inspiring others to switch to veganism involves approaching the topic with empathy, information, and a positive attitude. Here are some strategies to effectively encourage friends and family to consider a vegan lifestyle.

Be a shining example of a healthy, compassionate, and sustainable vegan lifestyle. When others see you thriving on a vegan diet and embracing the ethical and environmental aspects, they may be more inclined to follow suit. Equip yourself with knowledge about veganism, including the ethical, environmental, and health reasons for choosing this lifestyle. Being well-informed will enable you to answer questions and address concerns effectively. Initiate conversations about veganism by asking open-ended questions about their thoughts on animal welfare, health, or environmental issues. Be a good listener and genuinely understand their perspectives.

Share your personal journey toward veganism, including the reasons that motivated you to make the switch. Personal stories can be compelling and relatable. Provide books, documentaries, articles, and websites that offer information about veganism and its benefits. Encourage them to explore these resources at their own pace. Invite friends and family to try delicious vegan meals you've prepared. Host a vegan dinner party or cook vegan dishes for special occasions to show them how enjoyable and satisfying vegan food can be.

Emphasize the health benefits of a vegan diet, such as lower cholesterol, reduced risk of chronic diseases, and increased energy levels. Share success stories of individuals who have improved their health through veganism. Be prepared to address common concerns or misconceptions about veganism, such as protein intake, nutrient deficiencies, and the feasibility of a vegan lifestyle. Let your friends and family know that you're there to support them on their journey to veganism. Offer to help them find vegan recipes, meal ideas, or local vegan restaurants. Recognize that people may need time to make the transition to veganism. Be patient and avoid judgment. Encourage small steps and gradual changes. Encourage them to connect with local or online vegan communities where they can find support, ask questions, and share experiences.

Share stories of well-known individuals, athletes, and celebrities who have embraced veganism. Positive role models can inspire and influence others. Suggest starting with meatless days or incorporating Meatless Mondays into their routine. Gradual changes can be more manageable for some people. Celebrate their milestones and achievements along their vegan journey, no matter how small. Positive reinforcement can be motivating. Continue to gently introduce the topic of veganism over time, but always respect their choices and autonomy.

Remember that each person's journey to veganism is unique, and some individuals may need more time and information to make the switch. Your role is to provide support, resources, and inspiration, while ultimately allowing them to make their own decisions regarding their dietary choices.

Chapter 6: Resources

There are many excellent books, documentaries, and websites that can provide valuable information and resources for learning more about veganism. Here is a selection of some well-regarded ones in each category:

Books:

"Eating Animals" by Jonathan Safran Foer: This book explores the ethical, environmental, and health aspects of factory farming and the reasons to consider a vegan lifestyle.

"The China Study" by T. Colin Campbell and Thomas M. Campbell II: This comprehensive book delves into the health benefits of a plant-based diet, drawing on extensive scientific research.

"Animal Liberation" by Peter Singer: A seminal work in the animal rights movement, this book examines the moral and ethical arguments for animal rights and veganism.

"How to Create a Vegan World" by Tobias Leenaert: This book offers practical advice on effective vegan advocacy and how to communicate with non-vegans.

"Vegan for Life" by Jack Norris and Virginia Messina: A comprehensive guide to vegan nutrition, addressing common concerns and providing practical dietary advice.

Documentaries:

"Earthlings" (2005): A powerful and often difficult-to-watch documentary that explores the treatment of animals in various industries, making a compelling case for veganism.

"Cowspiracy: The Sustainability Secret" (2014): This documentary examines the environmental impact of animal agriculture and its role in climate change.

"Forks Over Knives" (2011): This film explores the health benefits of a whole-food, plant-based diet and features experts in the field of nutrition.

"Dominion" (2018): Similar to "Earthlings," this documentary provides an unflinching look at the treatment of animals in various industries.

"What the Health" (2017): This documentary investigates the health implications of consuming animal products and the influence of the pharmaceutical and food industries on public health.

Websites:

The Vegan Society: A comprehensive resource for all things vegan, including recipes, information on veganism, and advocacy opportunities.

HappyCow: A website and app that helps you find vegan and vegetarian restaurants, cafes, and stores in your area and around the world.

NutritionFacts.org: Dr. Michael Greger's website provides evidence-based information on nutrition and health, including topics related to veganism.

Plant Based News: A source for the latest news and articles related to veganism, plant-based diets, and animal rights.

VegNews: An online vegan lifestyle magazine that covers a wide range of topics, from recipes to news and trends.

These resources offer a wealth of information and different perspectives on veganism, making them valuable tools for those interested in learning more or deepening their understanding of this lifestyle.

Chapter 7: Sample Vegan Meal Plans

Plan #1

Breakfast: Vegan Breakfast Burrito

- Scrambled tofu with sautéed vegetables (bell peppers, onions, spinach) and turmeric for color and flavor.
- Black beans or pinto beans.
- Whole-grain tortilla or wrap.
- Top with avocado slices, salsa, and a sprinkle of nutritional yeast for a cheesy flavor.

Snack: Fresh Fruit Salad

- A mix of seasonal fresh fruits such as strawberries, blueberries, mango, and pineapple.
- Optional: A drizzle of lemon or lime juice and a pinch of mint leaves for extra freshness.

Lunch: Vegan Chickpea Salad

- Chickpeas (garbanzo beans) mixed with diced cucumbers, cherry tomatoes, red onions, and fresh parsley.
- Dress with olive oil, lemon juice, garlic, salt, and pepper.
- Serve over a bed of mixed greens or in a whole-grain pita.

Snack: Hummus and Veggie Sticks

- Baby carrots, cucumber slices, and bell pepper strips with a side of hummus for dipping.

Dinner: Vegan Stir-Fry

- Tofu or tempeh chunks stir-fried with broccoli florets, snap peas, bell peppers, and sliced mushrooms.
- Use a stir-fry sauce made from soy sauce, ginger, garlic, and a touch of agave or maple syrup.
- Serve over cooked brown rice or quinoa.

Dessert: Vegan Chocolate Avocado Mousse

- Blend ripe avocados, cocoa powder, a sweetener like agave or maple syrup, and a pinch of salt until creamy.

- Chill in the refrigerator before serving.

Note: Ensure you stay hydrated throughout the day by drinking water, herbal tea, or other non-dairy beverages. Also, consider taking a vitamin B12 supplement or including fortified foods in your diet to meet your nutritional needs.

This meal plan is just one example of a day of vegan eating, and there are countless other delicious and nutritious vegan meals you can enjoy. Feel free to modify it to suit your preferences and nutritional requirements.

Plan #2

Breakfast: Classic Vegan Pancakes

- Pancakes: Prepare fluffy vegan pancakes using a batter made from flour, almond milk, a touch of maple syrup, baking powder, and a pinch of salt.
- Toppings: Top your pancakes with sliced bananas, fresh berries, and a drizzle of pure maple syrup.
- Beverage: Enjoy a hot cup of black coffee or your favorite herbal tea.

Lunch: Quinoa and Vegetable Bowl

- Quinoa Bowl: Cook quinoa and top it with roasted or steamed vegetables (such as broccoli, cauliflower, and carrots).
- Protein: Add chickpeas or baked tofu cubes for protein.
- Sauce: Drizzle tahini or a homemade lemon-tahini dressing over the bowl.
- Side: Serve with a mixed green salad.

Snack: Peanut Butter and Banana Sandwich

- Sandwich: Spread natural peanut butter on whole-grain bread and add sliced bananas for a satisfying and quick snack.

Dinner: Vegan Lentil Soup

- Soup: Prepare a hearty lentil soup with red lentils, diced tomatoes, carrots, celery, onions, garlic, and vegetable broth.
- Seasoning: Season with cumin, coriander, and smoked paprika for depth of flavor.
- Serve: Garnish with fresh parsley and a squeeze of lemon juice.
- Side: Pair with a slice of crusty whole-grain bread.

Dessert: Vegan Fruit Salad

- Fruit Salad: Combine a variety of fresh fruits like strawberries, blueberries, kiwi, and orange segments in a bowl.
- Dressing: Drizzle with a light dressing made from maple syrup, lime juice, and a pinch of mint.

Plan #3

Breakfast: Avocado Toast

- Avocado Toast: Spread mashed avocado on whole-grain toast and sprinkle with red pepper flakes, salt, and a squeeze of fresh lemon juice.
- Toppings: Top with sliced cherry tomatoes and arugula.
- Beverage: Enjoy a cup of herbal tea or a dairy-free latte with almond milk.

Lunch: Vegan Mediterranean Salad

- Salad Base: Create a salad with a mix of greens, including romaine lettuce, arugula, and spinach.
- Veggies: Add diced cucumbers, red onion slices, Kalamata olives, and cherry tomatoes.
- Protein: Top with marinated and grilled tempeh or falafel.
- Dressing: Drizzle with a zesty lemon-tahini dressing.
- Side: Serve with a side of warm pita bread or whole-grain crackers.

Snack: Vegan Hummus and Veggie Sticks

- Hummus: Enjoy a generous serving of hummus made from chickpeas, tahini, lemon juice, garlic, and olive oil.
- Veggies: Dip baby carrots, celery sticks, and bell pepper strips into the hummus for a satisfying snack.

Dinner: Vegan Stir-Fried Tofu and Vegetables

- Stir-Fry: Sauté tofu cubes in a wok with a variety of colorful vegetables like broccoli, bell peppers, snap peas, and carrots.
- Sauce: Make a savory sauce with soy sauce, garlic, ginger, and a touch of agave nectar for sweetness.
- Grain: Serve the stir-fry over cooked brown rice or quinoa.
- Garnish: Top with chopped green onions and sesame seeds.
- Beverage: Enjoy a glass of water or sparkling water with a wedge of lime.

Vegan Stuffed Bell Peppers

These stuffed bell peppers are filled with a flavorful mixture of quinoa, black beans, corn, and spices, topped with a zesty tomato sauce. They make for an impressive and delicious dish for any special occasion.

Ingredients:

- 4 large bell peppers (any color)
- 1 cup cooked quinoa
- 1 can (15 oz) black beans, drained and rinsed
- 1 cup corn kernels (fresh, frozen, or canned)
- 1 small onion, finely chopped
- 2 cloves garlic, minced
- 1 teaspoon cumin
- 1 teaspoon chili powder
- Salt and pepper to taste
- 1 can (15 oz) tomato sauce
- 1/2 cup vegetable broth
- Fresh cilantro for garnish

Instructions:

Preheat your oven to 375°F (190°C).
Cut the tops off the bell peppers and remove the seeds and membranes. Rinse them and set them aside.
In a large skillet, sauté the chopped onion and garlic until translucent.
Add the cooked quinoa, black beans, corn, cumin, chili powder, salt, and pepper. Mix well.
In a separate bowl, mix the tomato sauce and vegetable broth.
Fill each bell pepper with the quinoa mixture, then place them in a baking dish.
Pour the tomato sauce mixture over the stuffed peppers.
Cover the dish with foil and bake for 30-35 minutes, or until the peppers are tender.
Garnish with fresh cilantro before serving.

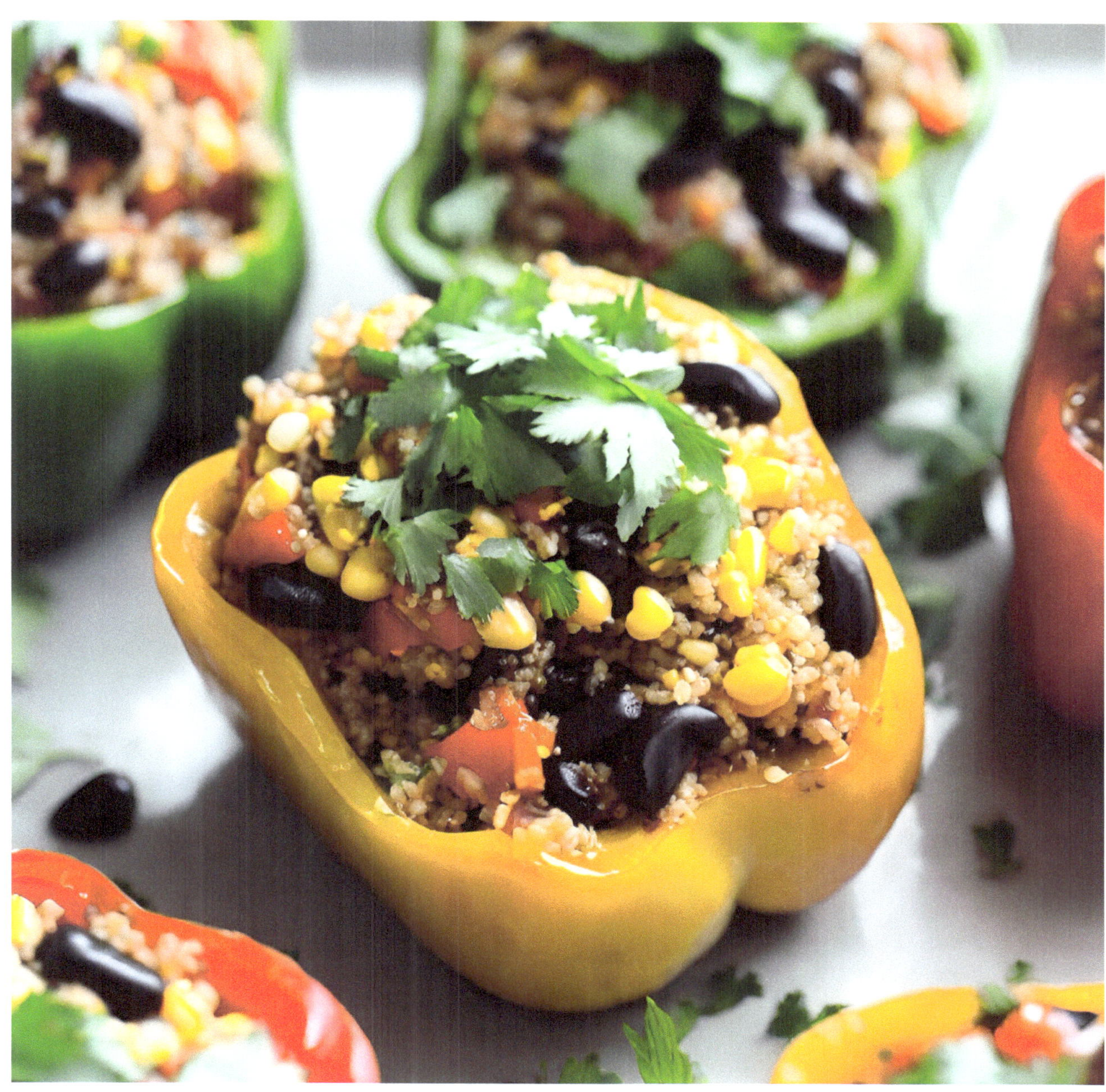

Vegan Mushroom Risotto

This creamy vegan mushroom risotto is rich and indulgent, making it perfect for special occasions.

Ingredients:

- 1 1/2 cups Arborio rice
- 8 oz (about 2 cups) cremini or button mushrooms, sliced
- 1 onion, finely chopped
- 2 cloves garlic, minced
- 4 cups vegetable broth
- 1 cup dry white wine (or vegetable broth for a non-alcoholic version)
- 2 tablespoons olive oil
- 1/2 cup nutritional yeast (for a cheesy flavor)
- Salt and black pepper to taste
- Fresh parsley for garnish

Instructions:

In a large pan, heat the olive oil over medium heat. Add the chopped onion and garlic, and sauté until translucent.

Add the sliced mushrooms and cook until they release their moisture and become browned.

Stir in the Arborio rice and cook for a couple of minutes until the rice is lightly toasted. Pour in the white wine and stir until it's mostly absorbed.

Begin adding the vegetable broth, one cup at a time, stirring frequently and allowing each cup to be absorbed before adding the next.

Continue to cook and stir until the rice is creamy and tender, which should take about 18-20 minutes.

Stir in the nutritional yeast for a cheesy flavor. Season with salt and black pepper to taste. Garnish with fresh parsley and serve hot.

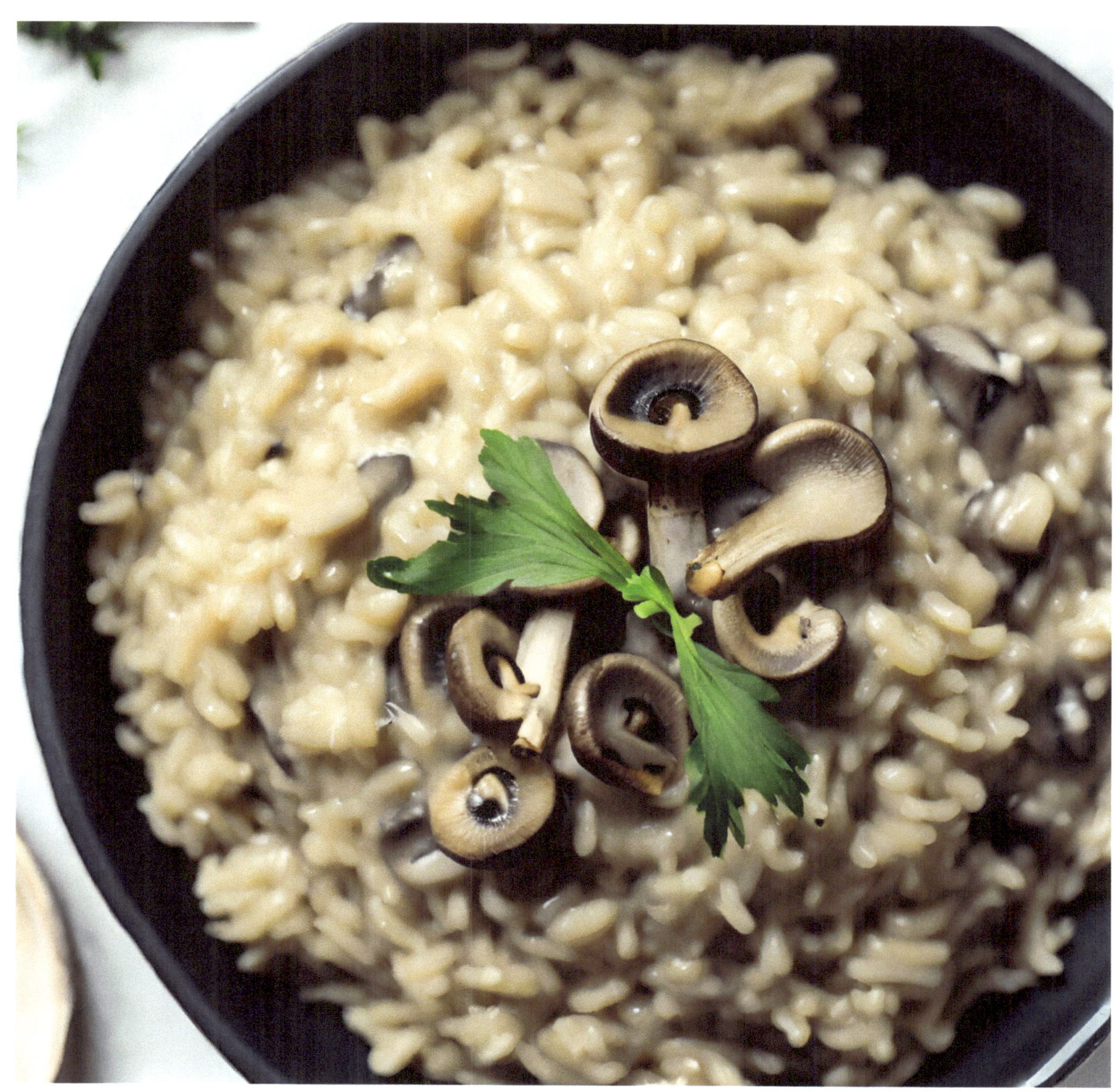

Vegan Chocolate Raspberry Tart

This vegan chocolate raspberry tart is a decadent dessert that's sure to impress your guests.

Ingredients:

For the Crust:

- 1 1/2 cups almond flour
- 1/4 cup cocoa powder
- 1/4 cup maple syrup
- 2 tablespoons coconut oil, melted

For the Filling:

- 1 1/2 cups dairy-free dark chocolate chips
- 1 cup full-fat coconut milk
- 1 teaspoon vanilla extract
- 1 1/2 cups fresh raspberries

Instructions:

For the Crust:

Preheat your oven to 350°F (175°C).
In a bowl, mix together almond flour, cocoa powder, maple syrup, and melted coconut oil until well combined.
Press the mixture into a tart pan to form the crust.
Bake the crust for 10-12 minutes, then let it cool.

For the Filling:

In a saucepan, heat the coconut milk until it starts to simmer. Remove from heat.
Add the dark chocolate chips and vanilla extract to the hot coconut milk. Stir until the chocolate is completely melted and the mixture is smooth.
Pour the chocolate filling into the cooled crust.
Arrange fresh raspberries on top of the chocolate filling.
Refrigerate the tart for at least 2 hours to set.
Before serving, you can dust the top with a little cocoa powder for decoration.

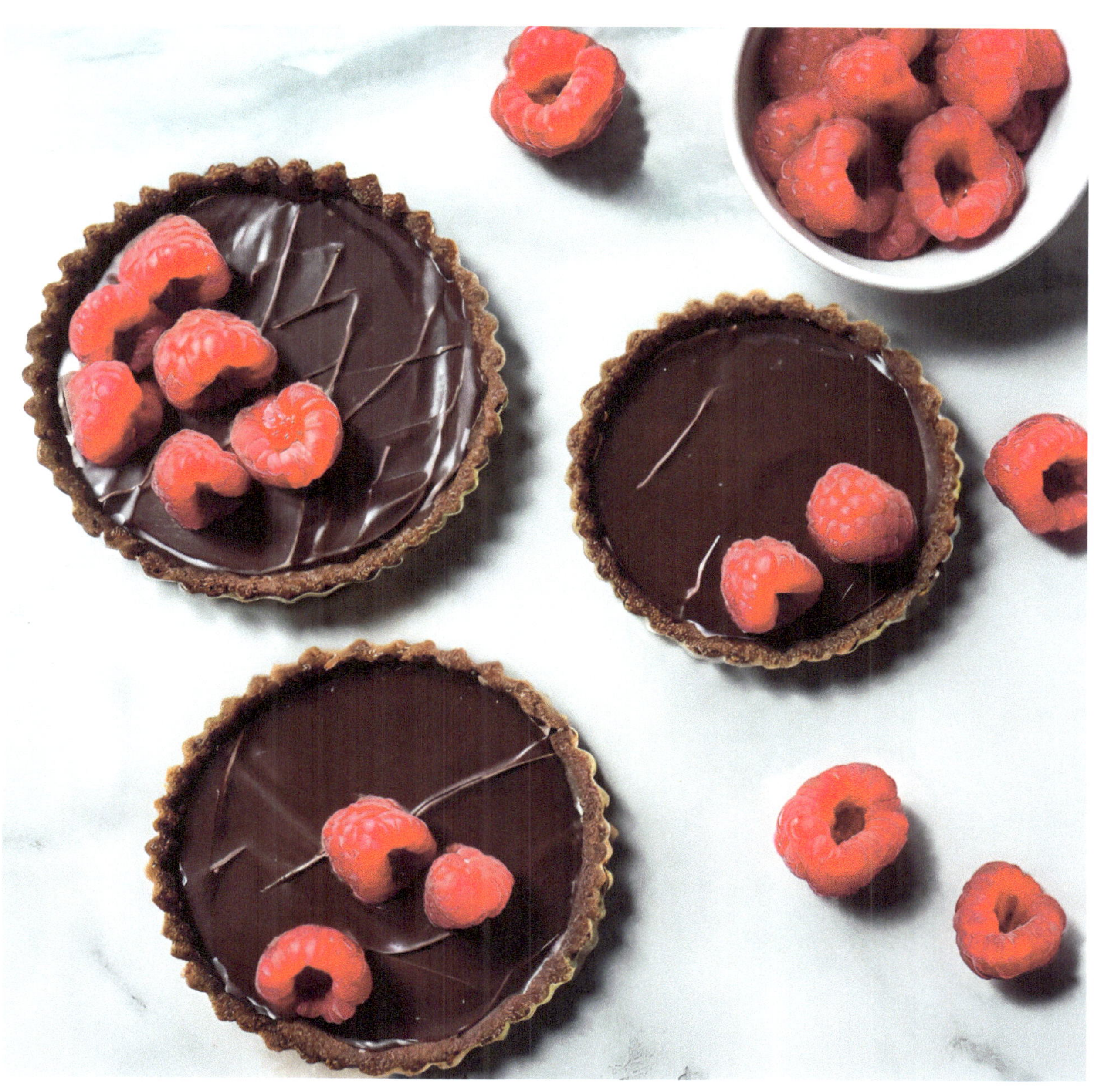

Vegan Chickpea Curry

This vegan chickpea curry is packed with flavor and protein, making it a satisfying and nutritious meal.

Ingredients:

- 1 tablespoon olive oil
- 1 onion, chopped
- 2 cloves garlic, minced
- 1-inch piece of ginger, grated
- 1 can (15 oz) chickpeas, drained and rinsed
- 1 can (14 oz) diced tomatoes
- 1 can (14 oz) coconut milk
- 2 teaspoons curry powder
- 1 teaspoon turmeric
- 1 teaspoon cumin
- 1 teaspoon paprika
- Salt and pepper to taste
- Fresh cilantro for garnish
- Cooked rice or naan bread for serving

Instructions:

In a large skillet, heat the olive oil over medium heat. Add the chopped onion and sauté until translucent.

Add the minced garlic and grated ginger. Sauté for another minute until fragrant.

Stir in the curry powder, turmeric, cumin, and paprika. Cook for a minute to toast the spices.

Add the chickpeas, diced tomatoes, and coconut milk. Stir to combine.

Season with salt and pepper to taste.

Simmer the curry on low heat for about 15-20 minutes, or until it thickens and the flavors meld together.

Serve the chickpea curry over cooked rice or with naan bread.

Garnish with fresh cilantro leaves before serving.

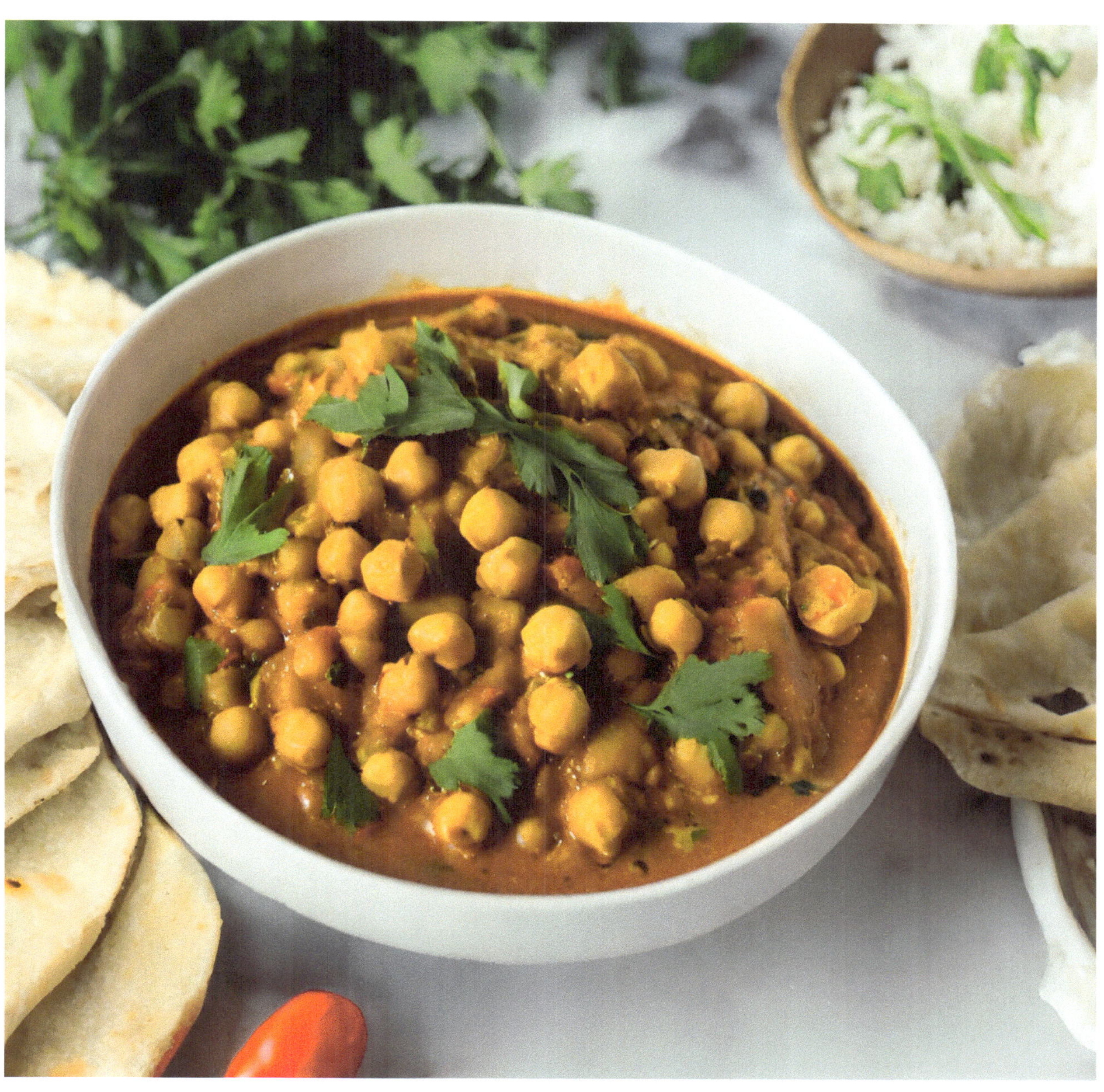

Vegan Mediterranean Quinoa Salad

adThis Mediterranean-inspired quinoa salad is loaded with fresh vegetables, olives, and a zesty lemon-tahini dressing.

Ingredients:

For the Salad:

- 1 cup quinoa, rinsed and cooked according to package instructions
- 1 cup cherry tomatoes, halved
- 1 cucumber, diced
- 1/2 red onion, finely chopped
- 1/2 cup Kalamata olives, pitted and sliced
- 1/2 cup fresh parsley, chopped
- 1/4 cup fresh mint leaves, chopped
- 1/4 cup toasted pine nuts (optional)

For the Dressing:

- 3 tablespoons tahini
- Juice of 1 lemon
- 2 tablespoons extra-virgin olive oil
- 2 cloves garlic, minced
- Salt and black pepper to taste
- Water (to thin, as needed)

Instructions:

In a large bowl, combine the cooked quinoa, cherry tomatoes, cucumber, red onion, Kalamata olives, parsley, mint, and pine nuts (if using).
In a separate small bowl, whisk together the tahini, lemon juice, extra-virgin olive oil, minced garlic, salt, and black pepper. If the dressing is too thick, you can add a little water to thin it out.
Drizzle the dressing over the salad and toss everything together until well coated.
Taste and adjust the seasoning if needed.
Refrigerate the salad for at least 30 minutes before serving to allow the flavors to meld together.
Serve as a main dish or as a side salad.

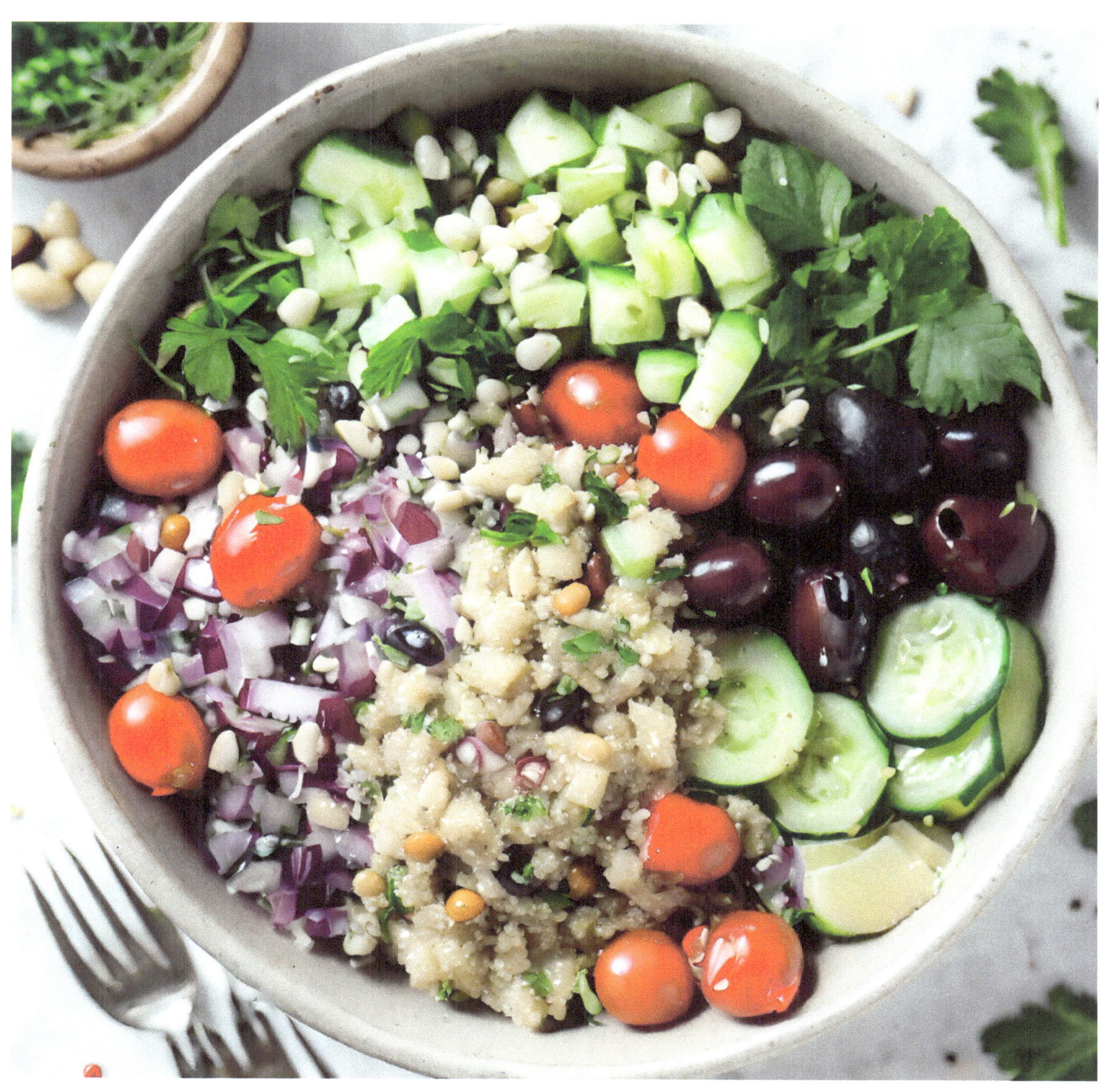

Chapter 8: Continuing Your Vegan Journey

Continuing a vegan lifestyle is not only commendable but also a decision that aligns with values of compassion, health, and sustainability. Reflect on the reasons that initially motivated you to go vegan. Whether it's for animal welfare, the environment, your health, or a combination of these, keeping your "why" in mind can be a powerful motivator. Take pride in the positive impact you're making. Every vegan meal, snack, or day contributes to reducing animal suffering and your carbon footprint. Celebrate your choices and their significance. Surround yourself with like-minded individuals. Join vegan groups, forums, or social media communities where you can share experiences, get support, and exchange ideas.

The vegan lifestyle offers a world of culinary adventure. Try new fruits, vegetables, grains, and plant-based products to keep your meals exciting and diverse. Continue to learn about veganism, nutrition, and the impact of your choices. Knowledge can reinforce your commitment and help you make informed decisions. If you're facing challenges, remember that it's okay to take small steps. Gradual changes can be more sustainable and less overwhelming. Being vegan doesn't mean you have to be perfect all the time. Occasionally, you may encounter situations where vegan options are limited. Do your best and adapt when necessary without guilt. Embrace the health benefits of a vegan diet. Many people experience increased energy, improved digestion, and a reduced risk of chronic diseases. Prioritize your well-being.

Educate others about veganism and its benefits, but do so with empathy and patience. Your positive influence can inspire others to make compassionate choices. Experiment with vegan cooking and try out new recipes. You might discover a passion for culinary creativity and enjoy making delicious vegan meals. Don't be too hard on yourself if you make occasional slip-ups or face challenges. Remember that it's a journey, and perfection is not the goal. Your commitment to a vegan lifestyle contributes to a more sustainable and compassionate world. Visualize the positive impact you're creating for future generations.

Keep up to date with developments in vegan products, restaurants, and initiatives. The growing availability of vegan options makes it easier than ever to stay vegan. Follow vegan influencers, watch documentaries, and read books and articles related to veganism to stay inspired and connected to the movement.

Remember that your choice to live a vegan lifestyle is meaningful and has a positive impact. Stay committed, and know that you are part of a global community working towards a more compassionate and sustainable world.

Appendix - Glossary of Vegan Terms

Vegan: A person who follows a lifestyle and diet that excludes all animal products, including meat, dairy, eggs, and honey, as well as non-food items like leather and fur.

Plant-Based: A term often used interchangeably with vegan, but it may refer specifically to a diet based on plants while not necessarily incorporating the broader lifestyle aspects of veganism.

Cruelty-Free: Products or practices that do not involve harming or testing on animals. This term is often used in reference to cosmetics, personal care items, and household products.

Ethical Vegan: Someone who adopts a vegan lifestyle primarily due to ethical concerns about animal exploitation and cruelty.

Dietary Vegan: A person who follows a vegan diet but may not fully embrace the ethical and lifestyle aspects of veganism.

Whole Foods Plant-Based Diet: A diet focused on whole, minimally processed plant foods like fruits, vegetables, grains, legumes, nuts, and seeds, with an emphasis on health.

Raw Vegan: A vegan diet that consists primarily of raw, uncooked foods, often including fruits, vegetables, nuts, and seeds.

Nutritional Yeast: A deactivated yeast often used in vegan cooking to provide a cheesy or nutty flavor. It's a source of B vitamins and protein.

Tofu: A soy-based protein made from soybean curds. It has a neutral flavor and is used in a variety of dishes and cuisines.

Seitan: A protein-rich meat substitute made from wheat gluten. It has a chewy texture and is often used in vegan meat dishes.

Tempeh: A fermented soybean product with a nutty flavor and firm texture, high in protein and other nutrients.

Veggie Burger: A meatless burger typically made from ingredients like vegetables, legumes, grains, and spices.

Dairy Alternatives: Plant-based milk, cheese, and yogurt made from ingredients such as soy, almond, coconut, oats, or rice.

Aquafaba: The liquid from canned chickpeas or other legumes that can be whipped to create a vegan egg white substitute for baking.

Cruelty-Free Fashion: Clothing and accessories made without the use of animal-derived materials like leather, fur, and silk.

Plant Milk: Non-dairy milk made from plant sources such as almonds, soy, oats, or coconut.

Non-GMO: Products that do not contain genetically modified organisms.

Veganism Advocacy: Promoting the principles of veganism, including ethical, environmental, and health reasons, to raise awareness and encourage others to adopt a vegan lifestyle.

Veganuary: A campaign encouraging people to try veganism for the month of January.

Meatless Monday: A global movement promoting one day a week where individuals and institutions choose not to consume meat.

Flexitarian: Someone who primarily follows a vegetarian or vegan diet but occasionally consumes animal products.

Vegan Outreach: Educational programs and initiatives aimed at spreading information about veganism and its benefits.

Egg Replacer: Plant-based alternatives used in baking to replace eggs, such as flaxseeds, chia seeds, applesauce, or commercial egg replacers.

Vegan Certification: Labels and symbols on products indicating they are vegan-friendly and meet specific vegan standards.

VegFest: Festivals and events celebrating veganism, featuring vegan food vendors, speakers, and educational activities.